Pocket Guide
to Musculoskeletal
Diagnosis

D1460143

Pocket Guide to Musculoskeletal Diagnosis

By

Grant Cooper, MD

Department of Physical Medicine and Rehabilitation
New York Presbyterian Hospital, The University Hospitals
of Columbia and Cornell, New York, NY

Foreword by

Robert S. Gotlin, DO

Director, Orthopaedic and Sports Rehabilitation
Director, Sports and Spine Rehabilitation Fellowship Program
Beth Israel Medical Center, New York, NY

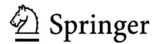 Springer

Editor
Grant Cooper, MD
Department of Physical Medicine
and Rehabilitation New York Presbyterian Hospital,
The University Hospitals of Columbia and Cornell,
New York, NY

Additional material to this book can be downloaded from http://extras.springer.comt

ISBN 978-1-58829-674-0   e-ISBN 978-1-59745-009-6
DOI 10.1007/978-1-59745-009-6

Cover illustration: From Figs. 3 and 12 in Chapter 1, "Neck and Shooting Arm Pain"
an Fig. 7 in Chapter 7, "Ankle Pain."
Cover design: Patricia F. Cleary

Printed on acid-free paper

springer.com

Dedication

*I dedicate this book to my mother, father, brothers, and to
the 6-second game—may we always remember to play.
And to Ana, what a wonderful adventure we're on...*

—G.C.

Foreword

The many musculoskeletal dilemmas faced by the health care practitioner on a daily basis challenge the caregiver to provide the most appropriate therapeutic intervention. Advances in medical research have stuffed the practitioner's medicine bag with a myriad of treatment options. As a result, statistically significant successful outcomes continue to increase in frequency. The new millennium has brought heightened public attention to and awareness of physical fitness and general well-being. Many are increasingly diet conscious, others pay close attention to workout schedules, and the majority of people enjoy a lengthened life expectancy.

Apace with the fitness craze, the medical profession continues to see a rise in musculoskeletal injuries. Although most—such as sprains and strains—are minor, others are more significant, including fractures and head injuries. The common denominator in evaluating and treating these maladies is the establishment of a clear and precise working diagnosis. When the health care practitioner has resources available to derive the working diagnosis, the ensuing work-up is simplified.

The *Pocket Guide to Musculoskeletal Diagnosis* is just such a resource. Author Grant Cooper has systematically written a practical guide to assist the medical clinician in establishing a working diagnosis, and he offers appropriate work-up and treatment options for many musculoskeletal ailments. The guide is sectioned by body region and maintains superb clarity, consistency, and organization in its writing. This comprehensive guide allows the busy practitioner to have at hand a resource that raises awareness not only of specific diagnoses, but also associated maladies inclusive in the differential diagnosis.

This guide is one I will recommend not only to young physicians in training, but also to my peers and colleagues.

Robert S. Gotlin, DO
Director, Orthopaedic & Sports Rehabilitation
Director, Sports and Spine Rehabilitation Fellowship Program
Beth Israel Medical Center
New York, NY

Preface

As a student and teacher of medicine, I have always appreciated books that slice through the extraneous material and get to the heart of the matter. In musculoskeletal medicine, there are few books that accomplish this task. As I sat down to write *Pocket Guide to Musculoskeletal Diagnosis*, I began to appreciate the reason for this paucity. Invariably, when you filter information, material will be left out that someone thinks is important. In consideration of that fact, we often permit ourselves, and even unwittingly may encourage ourselves, to become sidetracked into the minutiae. Of course, minutia has its place and is critical to appreciate. But it doesn't have a place in a high-yield book. In *Pocket Guide to Musculoskeletal Diagnosis*, I have tried to distill the information into a concise, easily digestible book intended for comprehensive, but also rapid, study.

After reading this book, I hope you will feel comfortable performing a history and physical examination for musculoskeletal problems. In addition, it is my hope that you will appreciate the basic pathophysiology of the most common musculoskeletal disorders, and gain some additional insight into the common misconceptions surrounding these disorders. For instance, the diagnoses of radiculopathy, radicular pain, referred pain, and nociceptive pain are often confused, misunderstood, and inappropriately managed. *Pocket Guide to Musculoskeletal Diagnosis* addresses these issues and their implications in what I hope you will find is a clear, pragmatic style.

I encourage you to think of *Pocket Guide to Musculoskeletal Diagnosis* as "easy-reading" and to use it to guide your approach to the musculoskeletal complaint. For more in-depth study, it would be appropriate to reference a more detailed text, of which there are many good ones. I hope you enjoy reading this book as much as I enjoyed writing it.

Grant Cooper, MD

Acknowledgments

This book is the product of a terrific collaborative effort and it is my privilege to take a few lines to acknowledge the many people involved. First, I would like to extend a special thank you to Don Odom and Humana Press. Don Odom's vision and unwavering support for this book helped make it a reality. Thank you also to Damien DeFrances, a wonderful editor and great help with this book. Brian Kao was the photographer for the pictures in this book and did a superb job. His work can be found at www.CaptureYourself.com. Paul Bree edited the pictures and also did an outstanding job. Finally, I would be remiss not to mention my early mentors for helping to form my own outlook on the approach to the musculoskeletal complaint. We all have mentors who make special impressions on us. These are some of mine: Nikolai Bogduk, PhD, DSc, MD; Paul M. Cooke, MD; Robert S. Gotlin, MD; and Gregory E. Lutz, MD.

—G.C.

Contents

1 Neck and Shooting Arm Pain

First Thoughts and Basic (and a Little Not-So-Basic) Pathophysiology

The pathological processes underlying complaints of neck and shooting arm pain often reside within the cervical spine. Therefore, essentially, the same physical examination is performed for both complaints. It is important to remember, however, that the diagnostic and therapeutic approach to neck pain is very different from that for shooting arm pain. This point will be discussed in greater detail in the section entitled "Plan" in this chapter. However, it is important to appreciate that distinguishing axial neck pain from shooting arm pain during your history and physical examination is critical. Luckily, this is easily accomplished.

Before discussing the specific steps to take while performing the exam, let's briefly review the terminologies and pathophysiologies of axial neck and radicular pain. We need to understand the language of neck pain because confusing the terminologies may lead to misdiagnosis, which in turn leads to inappropriate treatment.

Shooting arm pain may be termed *radicular pain*. Radicular pain is lancinating or electric in nature. Radicular pain radiates deeply in a narrow, characteristic, band-like pattern. The pathological mechanism of radicular pain is compression of a dorsal root ganglion or inflammation of a nerve root. Radicular pain and radiculopathy often (though not always) coexist. Radiculopathy is a neurological condition of loss—a sensory radiculopathy results in loss of sensation (numbness or tingling); a motor radiculopathy results in loss of strength (weakness). Loss of reflexes may result from a sensory, motor, or mixed radiculopathy. (**Note:** a sensory radiculopathy involves numbness or tingling, *not* pain.)

From: *Pocket Guide to Musculoskeletal Diagnosis*
G. Cooper

Radiculopathy is caused by ischemia or compression of nerve roots. Because radicular pain and radiculopathy often coexist, and because their evaluation and treatment are essentially equivalent, for the purposes of this book the two entities will be considered together. Common causes of radicular symptoms in the neck include cervical disc herniation (most common), disc osteophytes, zygapophysial (Z)-joint hypertrophy, and other various causes of spinal stenosis.

Axial neck pain is termed *nociceptive pain*. Nociceptive pain arises as a result of direct stimulation of nerve endings within the structure that is also the source of pain. Axial neck pain is perceived as dull and aching, and is often accompanied by referred pain (referred pain is perceived in a region other than the pathological source of pain). Whereas axial neck pain is caused by a structure within the neck and perceived in the neck, referred pain from the neck is caused by a structure within the neck but is perceived in a different location—for example, the head or arm. Referred pain is perceived as dull, aching, deep, and difficult to localize. When the pathological source of pain is within the cervical spine, referral pain patterns have consistently been found to include the head, shoulder, scapula, and/or arm.

The pathophysiology of referred pain is based on the principle of convergence within the central nervous system. In convergence, the afferent nerve fibers from two separate sites converge higher in the central nervous system. The brain then has trouble distinguishing the original source of pain, and so pain is perceived in multiple areas. In the neck, for example, a patient with Z-joint disease may present with dull axial pain in the neck and a referral pain pattern in the head, scapula, or arm that is aching and difficult to precisely localize.

Acute axial neck pain has been attributed to many potential causes, including somewhat ambiguous diagnoses, such as "muscle strain" and "whiplash." The truth is that we really do not know for sure what causes most cases of acute neck pain. This absence of data is owing in part to the fact that most cases of acute axial neck pain resolve without treatment. Therefore, aggressive diagnosis of the underlying cause is usually not warranted.

When acute neck pain lasts longer than 3 months, we call it *chronic neck pain*. Chronic neck pain is less likely to spontaneously resolve, and therefore merits more careful investigation. The most common cause of chronic neck pain has been shown to be cervical Z-joint disease. The Z-joints are the facet joints that articulate the inferior articular processes of one vertebra with the superior articular processes of the adjacent inferior vertebra. When a history of whiplash is elicited, Z-joint disease accounts for as much as 50% of cases of chronic neck pain, and up to 80% of cases of chronic neck pain following high-speed motor vehicle accidents, in particular. Other causes to consider in the differential diagnosis of chronic neck pain include osteoarthritis, discogenic pain, rheumatoid arthritis, and fracture.

Table 1
Axial, Referred, and Radicular Pain, and Radiculopathy

Pain	Characteristics	Pathophysiology
Axial pain	Dull, deep, aching, localized	Stimulation of the nerve endings within the structure that is also the source of pain.
Referred pain	Dull, deep, aching, and difficult to localize	The brain has difficulty distinguishing the true source of pain when afferent nerve fibers from two separate sites converge, and so pain is perceived vaguely in multiple areas.
Radicular pain	Lancinating, shooting, electric, band-like.	Compression of a dorsal root ganglion or inflammation of a nerve root.
Radiculopathy	Weakness, numbness, tingling, decreased reflexes	Ischemia or compression of a nerve root.

History

Ask your patient the following questions:

1. Where is your pain?

The location of your patient's pain is very important. Pain that stays within the neck is likely to be axial neck pain. Pain that is diffuse and difficult to localize is more likely to be axial neck pain with a referral pain pattern. Band-like pain is more likely to be radicular pain. Radicular symptoms in the lateral shoulder and lateral antecubital fossa are most often associated with the C5 nerve root. Radicular symptoms in the first digit are most often associated with the C6 nerve root; radicular symptoms in the third digit are associated with the C7 nerve root; radicular symptoms in the fifth digit are associated with the C8 nerve root; and radicular symptoms in the medial antecubital fossa are associated with the T1 nerve root (Photo 1). Referred patterns of pain may occur in the head, scapula, and arm. Further questioning will help differentiate radicular pain from referred or axial nociceptive pain.

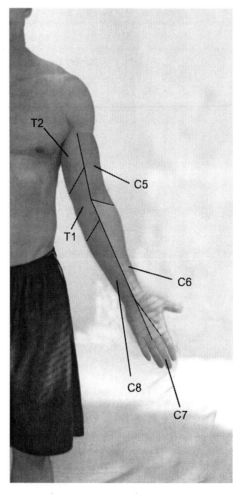

Photo 1. C5–T2 dermatomes.

2. What is the quality of your pain (i.e., dull, sharp, electric, radiating, or lancinating)?

This is the single most important question in differentiating axial from radicular pain. Radicular pain is *electric, lancinating, and shooting*. Axial and referred pain patterns are deep, aching, and/or sharp. Whereas radicular pain in the neck may *sometimes* present as dull or aching, axial and referred pain patterns are *never* lancinating, electric, or radiating.

3. When did your symptoms begin and what were you doing at the time?

This question is important for two reasons: first, if your patient's pain has lasted less than 3 months (acute pain), it is much more likely to resolve on its own. Second, patients with axial neck pain and a history of a motor vehicle accident immediately precipitating their symptoms have up to an 80% chance of their pain resulting from a diseased Z-joint. Patients with axial neck pain (with or without a referral pain pattern) and a history of neck trauma other than a motor vehicle accident precipitating their symptoms also have an increased probability of Z-joint disease causing their pain. A history of trauma precipitating acute (or chronic) neck pain necessitates ruling out the possibility of a fracture with X-ray and/or computed tomography evaluation in most cases.

4. Have you ever had a history of trauma to your head (i.e., a motor vehicle accident, being punched in the head)?

This question again focuses on Z-joint disease and axial neck pain. Most patients with Z-joint disease can recall some history of trauma (even if it was 60 years ago and did not immediately precipitate their symptoms).

5. Are there any positions that make your symptoms better or worse?

Patients with radicular symptoms caused by a herniated disc may be more likely to have worsening symptoms with neck flexion (which increases intradiscal pressure). Patients with radicular symptoms caused by foraminal stenosis may be more likely to have increased symptoms with neck oblique extension (such as looking back over the shoulder) because this position increases pressure on the foramen. Patients with Z-joint disease may have increased pain with neck extension because this position increases pressure on the Z-joints.

6. **Have you tried anything to help your pain?**

   This question is most helpful for deciding which imaging studies (if any) to order and how to treat your patient.

7. **Have you had any fevers, pain at rest, or night-time pain?**

   If the answer to any of these questions is "yes," then you should consider an underlying infection or malignancy.

8. **Have you been experiencing increasing weakness or numbness?**

   Progressive neurological injury is an indication for surgery and the patient should have spinal cord compromise ruled out.

Physical Exam

Having completed the history portion of your exam, you have determined whether or not your patient has symptoms of axial neck pain or radicular, and you have begun to narrow your differential diagnosis. It is now time to perform your physical exam. (**Note:** if a cervical fracture is suspected, obtain radiographs prior to performing a physical exam.)

Begin your exam with inspection. Observe any obvious asymmetry. Palpate the spinous processes. C7 is the largest cervical spinous process. To help differentiate C7 from T1, have the patient laterally rotate the head as you simultaneously palpate the spinous processes of C7 and T1. C7 will move slightly with lateral rotation but T1 is fixed and will not rotate. Palpate the paraspinal cervical muscles for any muscle spasms, tender points, or trigger points. Trigger points are differentiated from tender points because in addition to being tender, trigger points have referral pain patterns when palpated.

Next, assess the patient's range of motion. First, have the patient flex and extend the neck. Then have the patient rotate the head slowly from side to side (as if shaking the head "no"). Instruct the patient to laterally flex the neck (as if attempting to touch the ear to the ipsilateral shoulder). If the patient has limitations with active range of motion, assess passive range of motion by moving the head gently through the different movements.

Next, assess the patient's strength. Test the neck flexors by having the patient flex the head against resistance. This tests the sternocleidomastoid muscles, which are innervated by the spinal accessory nerve (cranial nerve XI).

Test the patient's neck extensors by having the patient extend the neck against resistance. This tests the paravertebral extensor muscles (splenius, semispinalis, and capitis), which are innervated by the dorsal rami from the segmental cervical nerve roots; and trapezius muscles, which are innervated by the spinal accessory nerve (cranial nerve XI).

Assess the patient's lateral rotation strength by having the patient laterally rotate the head against resistance. This tests the contralateral sternocleidomastoid muscle, which is innervated by the spinal accessory nerve (cranial nerve XI).

Test the patient's ability to laterally flex the head by having the patient attempt to touch the ear to the ipsilateral shoulder against resistance. This tests the ipsilateral sternocleidomastoid (innervated by cranial nerve XI) and scalaneus muscles, which are innervated by the ventral divisions of the lower cervical nerves.

Table 2 lists the movements of the neck, along with the involved muscles and their innervation.

Table 2
Primary Muscles and Innervation for Neck Movement

Movement	*Muscles*	*Innervation*
Neck flexion	Sternocleidomastoid	Spinal accessory nerve (cranial nerve XI)
Neck extension	1. Paravertebral extensors (splenius, semispinalis, and capitis muscles).	1. Dorsal rami of the segmental cervical nerve roots.
	2. Trapezius.	2. Spinal accessory nerve (cranial nerve XI).
Lateral rotation	Contralateral sternocleidomastoid muscle.	Spinal accessory nerve (cranial nerve XI).
Lateral flexion	1. Ipsilateral sternocleidomastoid muscle.	1. Spinal accessory nerve (cranial nerve XI).
	2. Scalaneus muscles.	2. Ventral division of the lower cervical nerves.

Test the integrity of the patient's nerve roots by assessing the motor function of the muscles. Have the patient abduct the arm against resistance (Photo 2). This tests the deltoid and supraspinatus muscles, which are innervated primarily by the C5 nerve root. Next, have the patient flex the elbow against resistance (Photo 3). This tests the biceps and brachialis, which are innervated by both C5 and C6. Have the patient

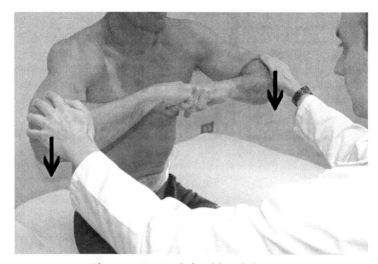

Photo 2. Resisted shoulder abduction.

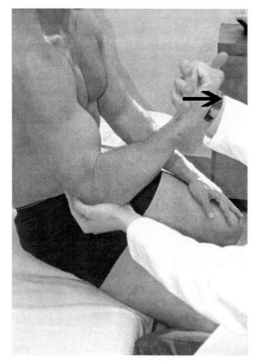

Photo 3. Resisted elbow flexion.

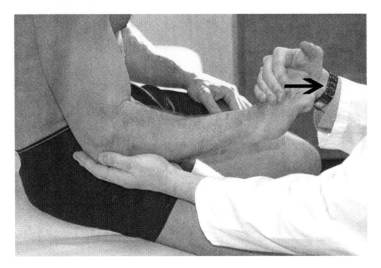

Photo 4. Resisted wrist extension.

then extend the wrist against resistance (Photo 4). This tests the patient's extensor carpi radialis longus and extensor carpi radialis brevis muscles, which are innervated by C6 and C7. Using the logic of reduction, the root of weakness can be determined. For example, if the patient has C6 weakness from C6 nerve root compression, then the patient's elbow flexion and wrist extension will be weak, but his or her shoulder abduction (C5) will be intact.

Next, have the patient extend the elbow against resistance (Photo 5). This tests the patient's triceps muscles, which are innervated by C7. Have the patient flex the fingers against resistance (Photo 6). This tests the patient's flexor digitorum superficialis (which flexes the proximal interphalangeal joint), and the patient's flexor digitorum profundus (which flexes the distal interphalangeal joint). Both of these muscles are innervated primarily by C8. Have the patient abduct and adduct the fingers (Photo 7). This tests the patient's interossei and abductor digiti minimi, which are innervated primarily by T1.

Table 3 lists the major movements of the arm, elbow, and hand, along with the involved muscles and their primary nerve root innervation.

Next, test the patient's sensation for any numbness or dysesthesia (abnormal sensation). Numbness or dysesthesia (as from a radiculopathy) will follow a dermatomal distribution. Check the patient's sensation

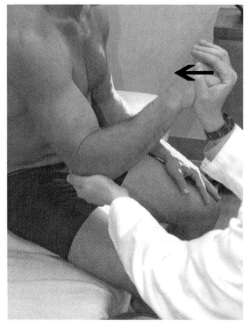

Photo 5. Resisted elbow extension.

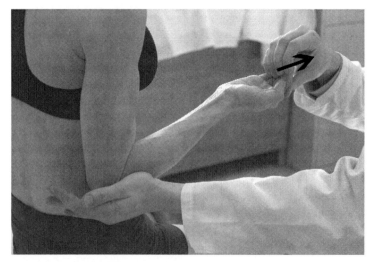

Photo 6. Resisted finger flexion.

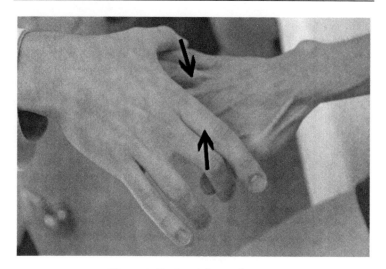

Photo 7. Resisted finger flexion.

Table 3

Primary Muscles and Root Level of Innervation for Shoulder, Arm, and Hand Movement

Major muscle movement	Primary muscles involved	Nerve root tested
Shoulder abduction	Supraspinatus and deltoid muscles	C5
Elbow flexion	Brachialis, biceps brachii	C6
Elbow extension	Triceps	C7
Finger flexion	Flexor digitorum superficialis and flexor digitorum profundus muscles	C8
Fifth-digit abduction	Abductor digiti minimi	T1

over the lateral antecubital fossa (C5), dorsal proximal phalanx of the first digit (C6), dorsal proximal phalanx of the third digit (C7), dorsal proximal phalanx of the fifth digit (C8), and medial antecubital fossa (T1) (Photo 8).

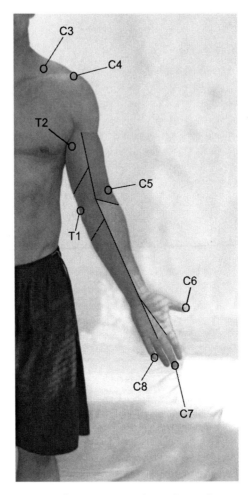

Photo 8. Upper dermatome with circles indicating locations to test. (Note that C6–C8 should be on the dorsal surface.)

Test the patient's reflexes: the biceps reflex (C5) (Photo 9), the brachioradialis reflex (C6) (Photo 10), and the triceps reflex (C7) (Photo 11).

Next, perform the Spurling's test. This test is used to assess foraminal stenosis. Perform this test by passively placing the patient's head into oblique extension in the direction of the affected side, and then

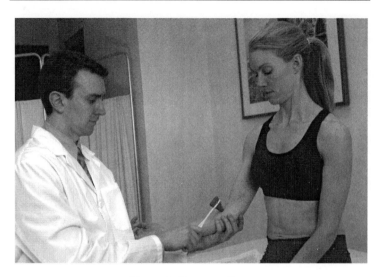

Photo 9. Biceps reflex.

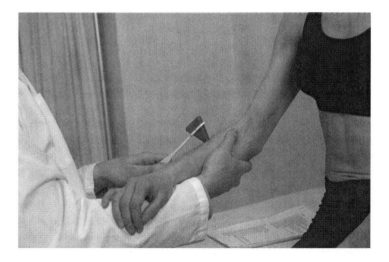

Photo 10. Brachioradialis reflex.

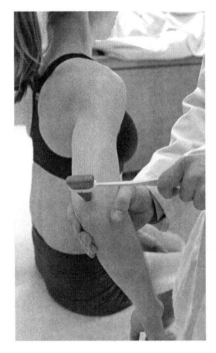
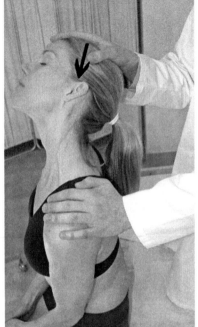

Photo 11. Triceps reflex.   Photo 12. Spurling's test.

applying gentle axial compression to the head (Photo 12). This maneuver introduces significant pressure onto the cervical foramen. If radicular symptoms down the arm are produced when this maneuver is performed, the patient has a positive Spurling's test, indicating foraminal stenosis.

Next, perform the distraction test. Perform this test by first returning the patient's head to the neutral position, and then placing one hand underneath the patient's chin and your other hand beneath the patient's occiput and lifting upwards (Photo 13). The distraction test is positive when it *relieves* the patient's pain; it works by *reducing* pressure on the foramen. When positive, the distraction test also indicates foraminal stenosis causing a radiculopathy.

Finally, test the patient to rule out an upper motor neuron lesion. This may be done by assessing for Hoffman's sign. To do so, hold the patient's third digit at the proximal interphalangeal joint and briskly

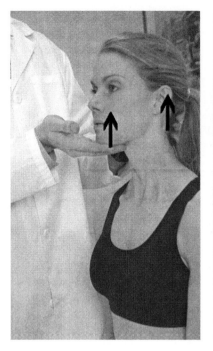

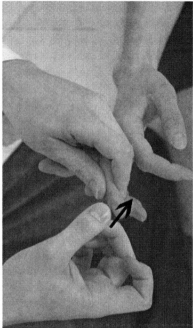

Photo 13. Distraction test.   Photo 14. Hoffman's sign.

flick the third distal phalanx (Photo 14). If the interphalangeal joint of
the thumb or the distal interphalangeal joint of the index finger of the
same hand flexes, the patient has a positive Hoffman's sign. The presence of hyperreflexia is also a sign of an upper motor neuron lesion.

Plan

Having completed the patient's history and physical examination,
you have a good idea of what is causing your patient's pain. Here is
what to do next:

- **Suspected Z-joint disease**

Additional diagnostic evaluation: There is no physical examination
technique or imaging study that can reliably diagnose Z-joint disease.
If your patient has chronic axial neck pain, X-rays or magnetic reso-

nance imaging (MRI) may be done to rule out more serious underlying pathology (such as fracture or tumor). However, only diagnostic blocks of the medial branches of the cervical dorsal rami innervating the suspected joint, or controlled intra-articular diagnostic blocks can diagnose cervical Z-joint disease (which is the most common cause of chronic axial neck pain with or without a referral pattern).

Treatment: Radiofrequency neurotomy of the medial branches of the dorsal rami innervating the painful joint(s). This is a percutaneous procedure performed under fluoroscopic guidance.

• Suspected cervical muscle strain

This diagnosis is generally reserved for cases of acute neck pain.

Additional diagnostic evaluation: Not generally indicated. X-ray—including anteroposterior (AP), lateral, and oblique views—is optional to rule out more serious underlying pathology.

Treatment: Conservative care, including physical therapy, nonsteroidal anti-inflammatory drugs (NSAIDs), heat, and trigger point or tender point injections, is usually effective in treating muscle strains. Patients may also benefit from wearing a neck collar while sleeping.

• Suspected cervical discogenic pain

Additional diagnostic evaluation: X-ray—including AP, lateral, and oblique views—to rule out a more serious underlying pathology is optional. MRI should be obtained. Provocative cervical discography should be performed and is the gold standard diagnosis of cervical discogenic pain. As this is an invasive procedure, it should only be performed when the index of suspicion is sufficiently high.

Treatment: Physical therapy, including stretching and strengthening exercises and heat, and NSAIDs are considered first-line treatment. Patients who do not respond to conservative therapy may require surgical intervention.

• Suspected cervical osteoarthritis

Additional diagnostic evaluation: X-ray—including AP and lateral views—is optional. Radiographic findings of cervical osteoarthritis do not reliably correlate with clinical symptoms and therefore, the value of X-rays is in ruling out more serious underlying pathology.

Treatment: Physical therapy, including stretching and strengthening exercises of the surrounding muscles. NSAIDs, rest, and an appropriate pillow for better neck support may also be helpful.

- **Suspected cervical radiculopathy**

Additional diagnostic evaluation: X-ray—including AP and lateral views—and MRI. Electrodiagnostic studies may also be helpful.

Treatment: Most cases of cervical radiculopathy respond very well to conservative care, including physical therapy, NSAIDs, and fluoroscopically guided epidural steroid injections. In refractory cases or severe cases with progressive neurological deficiencies (i.e., increasing weakness or numbness), surgery should be considered.

- **Suspected cervical myelopathy**

Cervical myelopathy results from cervical stenosis and is characterized by hand weakness, clumsiness, and occasional gait disturbances.

Additional diagnostic evaluation: X-ray—including AP and lateral views—may be obtained. However, MRI is the imaging modality of choice.

Treatment: Conservative care includes physical therapy, collar, NSAIDs, and fluoroscopically guided epidural steroid injections. Surgical decompression may be necessary depending on the severity of symptoms and the patient's response to more conservative interventions.

- **Suspected fracture**

More common cervical fractures include Jefferson fracture (burst fracture of the ring of C1), Hangman's fracture (traumatic spondylolisthesis of C2), odontoid fracture, Z-joint fractures, and spinous process fractures.

Imaging: X-ray, including AP, lateral, and odontoid views, and/or computed tomography or MRI.

Treatment: Neck immobilization with a collar or halo and/or possible surgery.

2 Shoulder Pain

First Thoughts

When your patient complains of "shoulder pain," your differential diagnosis of common causes includes the following four entities:

1. Impingement syndrome and rotator cuff disease.
2. Rotator cuff calcific tendonitis.
3. Biceps tendonitis.
4. Superior labral anterior posterior (SLAP) lesions.

Related complaints of stiffness or of the shoulder "giving way," expand your differential diagnosis to include adhesive capsulitis (frozen shoulder) and shoulder instability, respectively. A history of trauma expands the diagnosis to include acromioclavicular (AC) injury and fractures. A careful history and physical examination will narrow your differential diagnosis.

History

Ask the following questions:

1. Where is your pain?

Patients with rotator cuff tendonitis and rotator cuff calcific tendonitis will generally point directly beneath their acromion process. Patients with bicipital tendonitis will point slightly more distal along their arm over the bicipital sheath.

2. What movements, if any, exacerbate your pain?

This is a high-yield question for shoulder pain that should confirm your diagnosis. Patients with biceps tendonitis, rotator cuff tendonitis, or rotator cuff calcific tendonitis all complain of pain exacerbated by overhead movements. Patients with biceps tendonitis or SLAP lesions may complain of increased symptoms during deceleration movements (such as when pitching a baseball) in particular.

3. Does your shoulder ever give way?

Patients with shoulder instability will complain of their shoulder repeatedly "giving way."

4. Did your shoulder previously have pain, but is now only stiff?

This question specifically targets patients with adhesive capsulitis (frozen shoulder). Patients with adhesive capsulitis classically report a history of shoulder pain that gradually resolves and is replaced with stiffness.

5. How long have you had your shoulder pain and have you tried anything to help it?

These two questions are more useful for when you are ready to order imaging studies and decide treatment.

Physical Exam

Having completed the history portion of your examination, you are ready to perform the physical exam.

First, inspect for any obvious signs of muscle atrophy or asymmetry. Palpate the AC joint for any asymmetry or defect. Next, palpate along the biceps tendon as it runs in the bicipital groove (tenderness over a tendon may reflect tendonitis). To find the bicipital groove, palpate lateral to the coracoid process onto the lesser tuberosity of the humerus. Lateral to the lesser tuberosity is the bicipital groove. Have the patient slowly internally rotate the arm and you will feel your finger come out of the groove as the groove rotates. Next, palpate the subacromial bursa (located beneath the acromion). This is a common site of inflammation and impingement of the supraspinatus tendon. Palpate it by extending and internally rotating the arm. This exposes the bursa from under the acromion.

Assess the patient's range of motion by having the patient reach behind and across the back with one hand and touch the lower opposite scapula (Photo 1). This maneuver tests for internal rotation and adduction. Internal rotation and adduction may also be tested by having the patient reach across the chest and touch the opposite shoulder (Photo 2). Next, have the patient reach behind the neck and touch the opposite scapula (Photo 3). This is the Apley Scratch test, and it is used to assess for external rotation and abduction. Next, passively adduct the patient's arm across the chest (Photo 4). This maneuver stresses the AC joint and is used to assess for AC joint injury or arthritis.

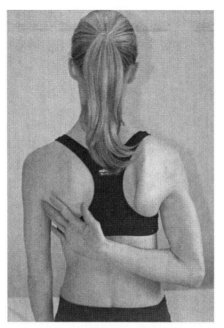

Photo 1. Apley Scratch test for shoulder internal rotation and abduction.

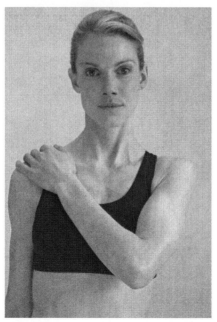

Photo 2. Shoulder internal rotation and adduction.

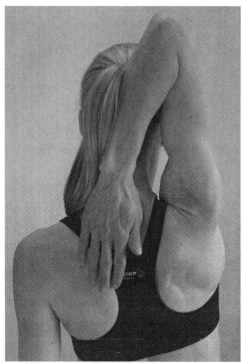

Photo 3. Apley Scratch test for external rotation and abduction.

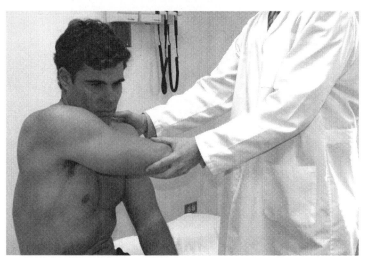

Photo 4. Passive cross arm test.

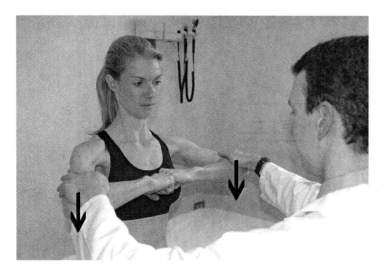

Photo 5. Resisted shoulder abduction.

Next, test the patient's shoulder strength. Test for shoulder flexion by having the patient flex the arm against resistance. This tests the anterior portion of the deltoid, which is innervated by the axillary nerve (C5), and the coracobrachialis (C5).

Test the patient's extension by having the patient extend the upper arm against resistance. This tests the latissimus dorsi, which is innervated by the thoracodorsal nerve (C6–C8); the teres major, which is innervated by the lower subscapular nerve (C5–C6); and the posterior portion of the patient's deltoid, which is innervated by the axillary nerve (C5–C6).

Test the patient's abduction by having the patient abduct the arm against resistance (Photo 5). This tests the middle portion of the deltoid, which is innervated by the axillary nerve (C5–C6); and the supraspinatus, which is innervated by the suprascapular nerve (C5–C6). The supraspinatus is primarily responsible for 0–30° of abduction. Therefore, it is important to test abduction by resisting the movement throughout its range of motion (or at least to 90°).

Test the patient's adduction by having the patient adduct the upper arm against resistance (Photo 6). This tests the patient's pectoralis major, which is innervated by the medial and lateral anterior thoracic nerves (C5–T1); the latissimus dorsi, which is innervated by the thoracodorsal

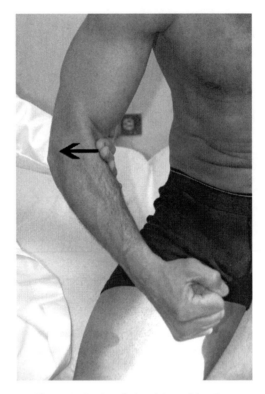

Photo 6. Resisted shoulder adduction.

nerve (C6–C8); and the teres major, which is innervated by the lower subscapular nerve (C5–C6).

Test the patient's external rotation by having the patient externally rotate the arm against resistance (Photo 7). This tests the infraspinatus muscle, which is innervated by the suprascapular nerve (C5–C6); and the teres minor, which is innervated by the axillary nerve (C5).

Test the patient's internal rotation by having the patient internally rotate against resistance (Photo 8). This tests the patient's subscapularis muscle, which is innervated by the upper and lower subscapular nerves (C5–C6); the pectoralis major muscle, which is innervated by the medial and lateral anterior thoracic nerves (C5–T1); the latissimus dorsi, which is innervated by the thoracodorsal nerve (C6–C8); and the teres major, which is innervated by the lower subscapular nerve (C5–C6).

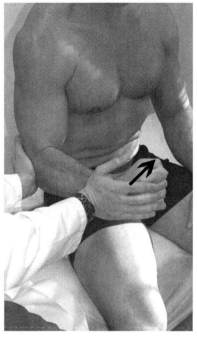
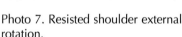
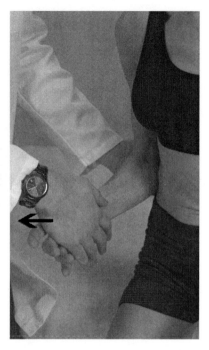

Photo 7. Resisted shoulder external rotation.

Photo 8. Resisted shoulder internal rotation.

Test the patient's scapular elevation by having the patient shrug his or her shoulders against resistance (Photo 9). This tests the patient's trapezius—which is innervated by the spinal accessory nerve (cranial nerve XI)—and the levator scapulae—which is innervated by branches of the dorsal scapular nerve (C5).

It is possible, although not routinely done, to test the patient's scapular retraction by having the patient stand "at attention" by throwing the shoulders back against the examiner's resistance. The examiner should provide resistance in this instance by trying to bend the patient's shoulders forward. This tests the patient's rhomboid major and minor muscles, both of which are innervated by the dorsal scapular nerve (C5).

Test for scapular protraction by having the patient push with two hands against a wall (Photo 10). This tests the patient's serratus anterior muscle, which is innervated by the long thoracic nerve (C5–C7). If the serratus anterior muscle is weak, medial scapular winging will be

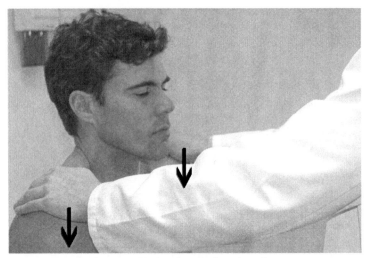

Photo 9. Resisted scapular elevation.

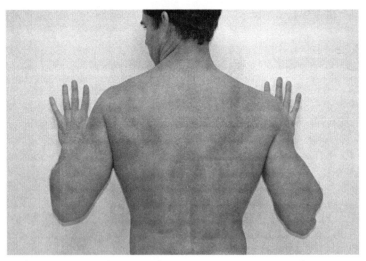

Photo 10. Test for scapular protraction. No scapular winging present.

evident. If the trapezius is weak, there may be lateral scapular winging evident.

Table 1 lists the movements of the shoulder, along with the involved muscles and their innervation.

Table 1
Primary Muscles and Root Level of Innervation
for Shoulder and Scapular Movement

Major muscle movement	*Primary muscles involved*	*Primary innervation*
Shoulder flexion	1. Anterior portion of the deltoid.	1. Axillary nerve (C5).
	2. Coracobrachialis.	2. Musculocutaneous nerve (C5,C6).
Shoulder extension	1. Latissimus dorsi.	1. Thoracodorsal nerve (C6–C8).
	2. Teres major.	2. Lower subscapular nerve (C5, C6).
	3. Posterior portion of the deltoid.	3. Axillary nerve (C5).
Internal rotation	1. Subscapularis.	1. Upper and lower nerves to the subscapularis (C5, C6).
	2. Pectoralis major.	2. Medial and lateral anterior thoracic nerves (C5–T1).
	3. Latissimus dorsi.	3. Thoracodorsal nerve (C6–C8).
	4. Teres major.	4. Lower subscapular nerve.
External rotation	1. Infraspinatus.	1. Suprascapular nerve (C5, C6).
	2. Teres minor.	2. Axillary nerve (C5).
Scapular elevation	1. Trapezius.	1. Spinal accessory nerve (cranial nerve XI).
	2. Levator scapulae.	2. Branches of the dorsal scapular nerve (C5).
Scapular retraction	1. Rhomboid major and minor muscles.	1. Dorsal scapular nerve (C5).
Scapular protraction	1. Serratus anterior muscle.	1. Long thoracic nerve (C5–C7).
	2. Trapezius.	2. Spinal accessory nerve (cranial nerve XI).

To test specifically for an anterior impingement syndrome, perform the Neer and Yocum tests. The Neer test is performed by internally rotating and passively flexing the patient's shoulder while keeping the arm in

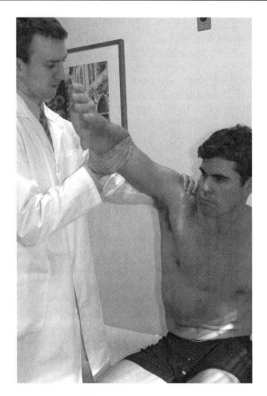

Photo 11. Neer test.

the scapular plane (Photo 11). This maneuver reduces the space between the acromion and greater tuberosity and may elicit pain in rotator cuff tendonitis. Pain is typically elicited at greater than 90° of flexion.

The Yocum test is a variation of the original Hawkins–Kennedy test. In the Yocum test, the patient's shoulder is abducted to 90°, and the elbow is flexed to about 60°. Using the hand and elbow as a fulcrum, the arm is forcibly put into internal rotation (Photo 12). This maneuver jams the supraspinatus tendon into the anterior surface of the coracoacromial ligament and acromion process. Pain is elicited in supraspinatus tendonitis.

When bicipital tendonitis is suspected, Speed's test is performed. In this test, the patient is instructed to supinate the arm, and the examiner resists the patient's shoulder flexion. The test is repeated with the

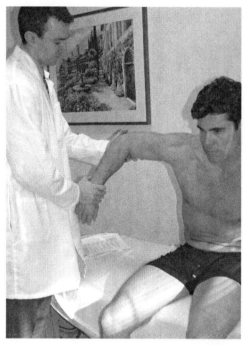

Photo 12. Yocum test.

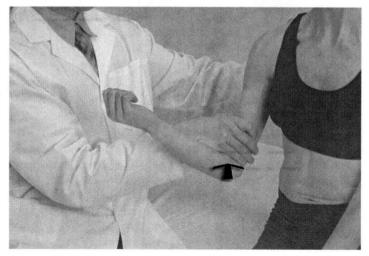

Photo 13. Speed's test.

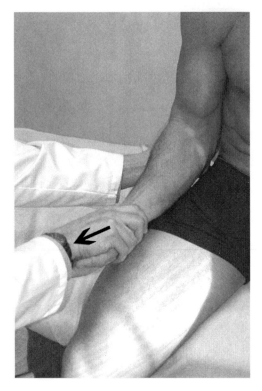

Photo 14. Yergason test.

patient's elbow flexed to 90° (Photo 13). The test is positive when pain
is elicited in the bicipital groove. The test may also be positive if a
SLAP lesion is present.

The Yergason test is also helpful in evaluating the biceps tendon. In
this test, the patient flexes the elbow to 90° while simultaneously internally rotating the shoulder and supinating the forearm against resistance. This test is positive and indicates a biceps injury if the maneuver
elicits pain over the long head of the biceps tendon (Photo 14).

To test more specifically for a SLAP lesion, and to differentiate it
from an AC joint injury, the O'Brien test is performed. In this test, the
patient stands with the shoulder flexed to 90° and the elbow in full
extension. The patient's shoulder is then put into 10–15° of adduction.
With the patient's hand supinated, the examiner puts an inferiorly
directed force on the patient's hand. The patient is then instructed to

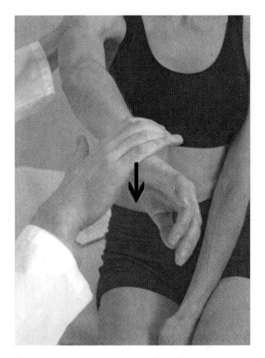

Photo 15. O'Brien test with hand in pronation.

fully pronate the hand (such that the thumbs are pointing down) and the examiner again places an inferiorly directed force onto the patient's forearm (Photo 15). When the maneuver elicits pain inside the shoulder when the hand is in pronation, but not when the hand is in supination, a SLAP lesion is suspected. However, this maneuver also stresses the AC joint. Therefore, if this maneuver elicits pain in the AC joint, pathology should be suspected in the AC joint and not in the labrum.

To test for a supraspinatus tear, perform the empty can test or the drop-arm test. To perform the empty can test, the patient is instructed to abduct the arm to 90° and flex the shoulder to 30°. The patient then internally rotates the arm so that the patient's thumbs are pointing down (as if emptying a can). Then the examiner pushes down (trying to adduct) the patient's arms (Photo 16). If there is weakness or pain with this maneuver, the patient may have a tear in the supraspinatus tendon or muscle, or a suprascapular neuropathy.

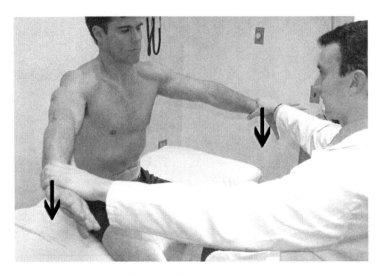

Photo 16. Empty can test.

To perform the drop-arm test, passively abduct the patient's shoulder to 90° and have the patient slowly lower the arm. If the patient is unable to slowly and smoothly lower the arm without pain, the patient may have a weak or torn supraspinatus tendon or muscle.

To test for subscapularis weakness, perform the Gerber lift-off test. In this test, the patient is instructed to put the hand behind the back with the dorsum of the hand against the lumbar spine. The patient is then instructed to push posteriorly against the examiner's resistance (Photo 17). Pain or weakness indicates subscapularis muscle or tendon weakness or injury. If the scapula shifts abnormally, this may reveal an underlying scapular instability.

To test for possible anterior instability, the apprehension test is performed. To perform this test, the patient's shoulder is passively abducted to 90° and the patient's elbow is flexed to 90°. The examiner then slowly externally rotates the patient's shoulder (Photo 18). If the patient appears apprehensive and resists this maneuver, the test is positive. It is important to perform this test slowly so as not to injure the patient by actually dislocating the shoulder. The apprehension test is then repeated, but this time, the examiner places additional posteriorly directed pressure onto the patient's anterior shoulder. By adding this posterior pressure, the patient should no longer be apprehensive with

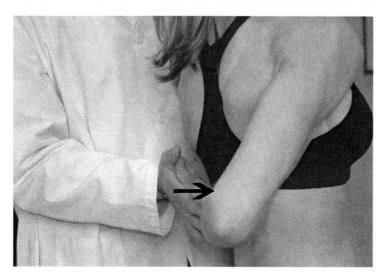

Photo 17. Gerber lift-off test.

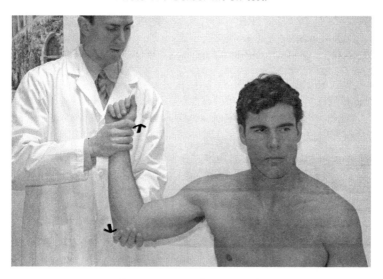

Photo 18. Apprehension test.

the maneuver (Photo 19). This is the relocation test and when it is positive, it confirms anterior shoulder instability. The apprehension test and the relocation test may be more easily performed with the patient in the supine position.

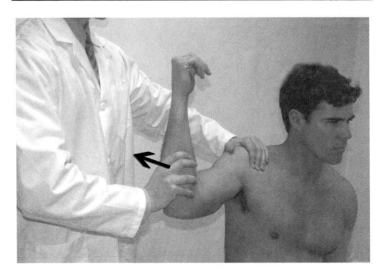

Photo 19. Relocation test.

Gross sensation testing should include the C3 dermatome, which is tested in the supraclavicular fossa; the C4 dermatome, which is tested over the AC joint; the axillary nerve, which is tested over the lateral aspect of the deltoid; and the C5 dermatome, which is tested over the lateral aspect of the elbow (Photo 20).

The biceps reflex (C5), brachioradialis reflex (C6), and triceps (C7) reflex should also be assessed as part of the physical examination of the shoulder.

Plan

Having completed your history and physical examination, you have a good idea of what is wrong with your patient's shoulder. Here is what to do next:

- **Suspected rotator cuff impingement syndrome**

Additional diagnostic evaluation: X-rays—including anteroposterior (AP) and lateral views of the shoulder in internal and external rotation, scapular outlet view, and axillary view—are often indicated. Magnetic resonance imaging (MRI) is generally not indicated unless a tear is suspected.

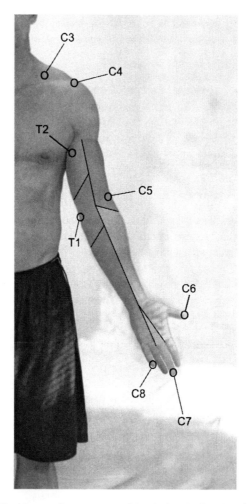

Photo 20. Upper dermatome with circles indicating locations to test. (Note that C6–C8 should be on the dorsal surface.)

Treatment: Conservative treatment is usually successful and includes rest, nonsteroidal anti-inflammatory drugs (NSAIDs), physical therapy, and/or a subacromial injection of corticosteroid and anesthetic. In the case of a calcification causing the tendonitis, ultrasound guided aspiration and lavage of the calcification has shown good results. Surgical treatment is reserved for refractory cases that have failed at least 3 months of conservative care.

- **Suspected subacromial bursitis**

  Additional diagnostic evaluation: X-rays—including AP and lateral views of the shoulder in internal and external rotation, scapular outlet view, and axillary view—are often obtained.

  Treatment: Conservative treatment, including rest, NSAIDs, physical therapy, and an injection of corticosteroid and anesthetic, is usually successful.

- **Suspected rotator cuff tear**

  Additional diagnostic evaluation: X-rays—including AP and lateral views of the shoulder in internal and external rotation, and axillary views—and MRI are indicated.

  Treatment: Conservative treatment, including physical therapy, is generally successful. Surgical repair for rotator cuff tears is reserved for partial tears refractory to conservative treatment and for full thickness tears.

- **Suspected bicipital tendonitis**

  Additional diagnostic evaluation: X-rays, including AP and lateral views of the shoulder in internal and external rotation, scapular outlet view, and axillary view, are often indicated.

  Treatment: Conservative treatment is usually successful and includes rest, NSAIDs, physical therapy, and/or a bicipital sheath injection of corticosteroid and anesthetic.

- **Suspected glenohumeral joint or acromioclavicular joint arthritis**

  Additional diagnostic evaluation: X-rays—including AP and lateral views of the shoulder, AP of the stressed (weights supported by the patient's wrists) and nonstressed AC joint, cephalic tilt, and scapular outlet view—are indicated.

  Treatment: Conservative treatment, including physical therapy, rest, NSAIDs, stretching, and strengthening exercises, is considered first-line treatment. An intra-articular corticosteroid and anesthetic injection may be helpful. Surgery is reserved for severe cases.

- **Suspected muscle strain**

  Additional diagnostic evaluation: none generally indicated.

Treatment: conservative treatment, including stretching and strengthening exercises, rest, and NSAIDs. Trigger point or tender point injections of anesthetic, normal saline, and steroids are often helpful.

- **Suspected adhesive capsulitis (frozen shoulder)**

Additional diagnostic evaluation: X-rays—including AP and lateral views of the shoulder in internal and external rotation, scapular outlet view, and axillary view—are generally indicated.

Treatment: Conservative treatment is usually successful and includes stretching and strengthening exercises, heat modalities, and NSAIDs. Intra-articular anesthetic and steroid injection may be particularly helpful early in the course of the pathology. Manipulation under anesthesia may also be helpful. Capsular release via either arthroscopic or open techniques is generally reserved for cases with severe and functionally limiting chronic symptoms.

- **Suspected shoulder instability:**

Additional diagnostic evaluation: X-rays—including AP and lateral views of the shoulder in internal and external rotation, scapular outlet view, and axillary view, computed tomography, and MRI—are indicated.

Treatment: Shoulder instability that is unilateral, precipitated by trauma, and accompanied by a Bankart lesion (a tear of the anterior glenoid labrum) is often treated with surgery. This may be remembered by the pneumonic TUBS—traumatic, unilateral, Bankart lesion, surgery. Shoulder instability that is multidirectional, bilateral, and not precipitated by trauma may often be treated with physical therapy, a sling, and/or inferior capsule repair. This may be remembered by the pneumonic AMBRI—atraumatic, multidirectional, bilateral, rehabilitation, inferior capsule repair.

- **Suspected SLAP lesion**

Additional diagnostic evaluation: X-rays—including AP and lateral views of the shoulder in internal and external rotation, scapular outlet, and axillary views—are indicated. MRI is indicated.

Treatment: Conservative care, including modification of activities and physical therapy, such as strengthening and stretching exercises, is the first-line treatment. Arthroscopic or open surgery is often necessary.

3   Elbow Pain

First Thoughts

When your patient complains of elbow or proximal forearm pain, your differential diagnosis of the most common causes includes lateral epicondylitis, medial epicondylitis, ulnar collateral ligament injury, fracture, rheumatoid arthritis, and cubital tunnel syndrome (in which the ulnar nerve is compressed at the cubital tunnel in the elbow). A careful history and physical examination will help narrow your differential.

History

Ask the following questions:

1. Where is your pain?

Patients with lateral epicondylitis will complain of pain over the lateral epicondyle. Patients with medial epicondylitis or ulnar collateral ligament injury will complain of pain over the medial elbow. Patients with cubital tunnel syndrome or ulnar collateral ligament injury may complain of a deep aching or electric sensation that may radiate from the elbow to their fourth and fifth digits.

2. What brought on the symptoms, and which movements most exacerbate them?

Patients with a history of trauma should be investigated for fractures. Humerus supracondylar fractures (most common in children), humerus intercondylar fractures (more common in adults), radial head fractures, and ulnar fractures are the more common fractures encountered.

Patients with an ulnar collateral ligament injury typically have pain that worsens with overhead activity. Patients with lateral

From: *Pocket Guide to Musculoskeletal Diagnosis*
G. Cooper

epicondylitis typically have pain that is worsened with activities that involve repetitive pronation and supination (e.g., tennis, throwing a ball, or plumbing). Patients with medial epicondylitis typically complain of pain that worsens with repetitive forearm pronation and wrist flexion, such as in golf.

3. **What is the quality of your pain—sharp, stabbing, numbness, tingling, etc.?**

   Patients with numbness, tingling, and shooting electric pains in the ulnar nerve distribution are likely to have cubital tunnel syndrome or ulnar collateral ligament injury (ulnar nerve symptoms are often associated with ulnar collateral ligament injury).

4. **Is the pain and swelling symmetrical?**

   This question is specifically for rheumatoid arthritis—a disease characterized in part by its symmetric distribution of symptoms.

5. **Have you noticed any weight loss or systemic symptoms, such as flushing or fever?**

   This question is also specifically for rheumatoid arthritis.

6. **Do you ever experience any locking or clicking in your elbow?**

   Patients with a loose body in their elbow from either a fracture or osteochondritis dissecans may complain of locking and/or clicking.

7. **Have you taken anything for the pain, and has it helped?**

   This question is more useful for when you are ready to order diagnostic studies and decide on treatment.

8. **Is there any grating when you move your elbow?**

   This question is specifically for osteoarthritis.

   Having completed the history portion of your examination, you have narrowed your differential diagnosis and are prepared to perform your physical exam.

Physical Exam

First, look for any swelling or asymmetry in the elbows. Patients with rheumatoid arthritis will have bilateral, symmetrical swelling. Palpate the joint as you move it passively through extension and flexion. Any crepitus may reflect underlying osteoarthritis or synovial or bursal thickening.

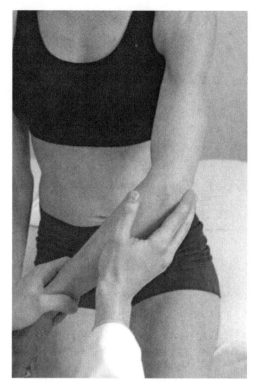

Photo 1. Olecranon bursa palpation.

Palpate posterior to the olecranon (Photo 1). There is a bursa in this location, and tenderness there indicates olecranon bursitis.

Next, palpate the medial collateral ligament, which attaches from the medial epicondyle of the humerus to the coronoid process and the olecranon of the ulna. This ligament is responsible for the medial stability of the elbow and is often injured in baseball pitchers because of the excessive valgus stresses placed on the ligament. Tenderness of the ligament indicates an underlying injury. Test for its stability by cupping the posterior aspect of the patient's elbow with one hand, and holding the patient's wrist with the other hand. Have the patient flex the elbow a few degrees and then apply a medially directed force to the patient's arm while simultaneously applying a laterally directed force to the patient's wrist. This maneuver places a valgus stress on the

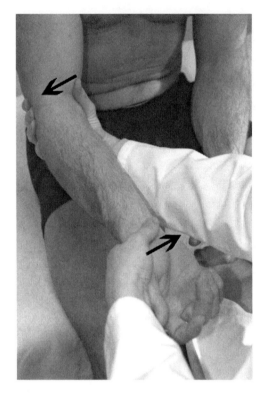

Photo 2. Varus stress to assess for lateral collateral injury.

patient's forearm. With the hand cupped under the patient's elbow, appreciate any medial gapping, which would indicate medial collateral ligament injury.

Next, palpate the lateral collateral ligament. Tenderness may indicate a lateral collateral ligament injury. Test the stability of the lateral collateral ligament by placing a varus stress on the forearm. Do this by placing a laterally directed force to the patient's arm and a medially directed force to the patient's wrist and note any gapping, which would indicate a lateral collateral ligament injury (Photo 2).

Palpate the ulnar nerve as it runs in the groove between the medial epicondyle and the olecranon (Photo 3). The ulnar nerve feels round and tubular, and you can roll it between your fingers. Tap the nerve repetitively. This is called "Tinel's sign." If repetitive tapping of the patient's

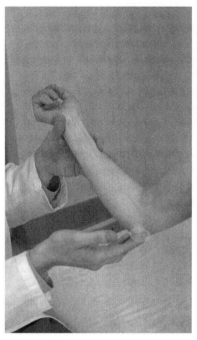 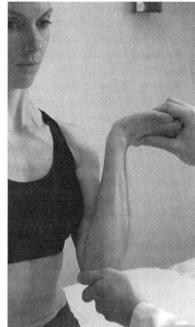

Photo 3. Ulnar nerve palpation.   Photo 4. Test for cubital tunnel
                                         syndrome.

ulnar nerve reproduces the patient's elbow pain and radiation of symptoms into the fourth and fifth digits, it is called a positive Tinel's sign,
and is indicative of cubital tunnel syndrome. However, because one-
quarter of asymptomatic people will have a positive Tinel's sign at this
location, it is a very nonspecific test. If cubital tunnel syndrome is suspected based on the patient's history, another test that may be performed
is to maximally flex the patient's elbow with the forearm supinated and
wrist extended (Photo 4). When this position is held for 60 seconds and
reproduces the patient's elbow pain and radiation of symptoms into the
fourth and fifth digits, it is considered a positive test for cubital tunnel
syndrome. However, this test is also nonspecific. Another clinical sign
for cubital tunnel syndrome is the Wartenberg sign. To elicit this sign,
passively spread the patient's fingers and instruct the patient to adduct
the fingers. Weakness or atrophy in the fifth digit adductor is a positive
Wartenberg sign.

Next, test for lateral epicondylitis. Start by palpating the lateral epicondyle of the patient's humerus for tenderness. After this, perform the Cozen test. To perform the Cozen test, the examiner stabilizes the patient's elbow with one hand and the patient is instructed to make a fist, pronate the forearm, and radially deviate the wrist. Finally, the patient is instructed to extend the wrist against resistance that is provided by the examiner (Photo 5). A positive Cozen's test is found if the patient experiences a sharp, sudden, severe pain over the lateral humeral epicondyle.

Now test for medial epicondylitis. First, palpate the medial epicondyle of the humerus. Then passively extend and supinate the elbow, and extend the wrist (Photo 6). When this maneuver elicits pain over the medial epicondyle of the humerus, the test is positive.

Next, test the patient's strength. Have the patient flex the elbow against resistance (Photo 7). This tests the patient's brachialis and biceps muscles, both of which are innervated by the musculocutaneous nerve (C5–C6).

Then have the patient extend the elbow against resistance (Photo 8). This tests the patient's triceps muscle, which is innervated by the radial nerve (C7).

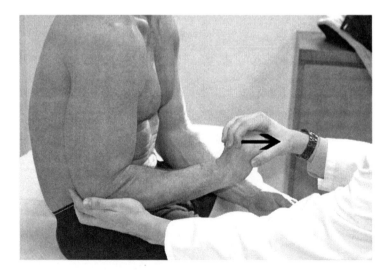

Photo 5. Cozen's test.

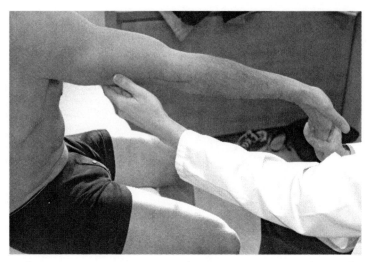

Photo 6. Passive extension and supination to assess for medial epidconylitis.

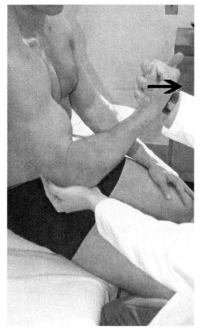

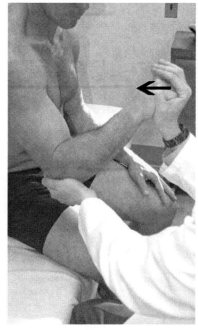

Photo 7. Resisted elbow flexion.   Photo 8. Resisted elbow extension.

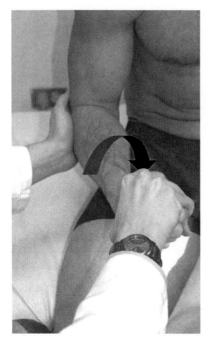 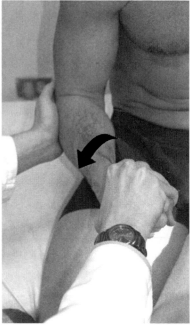

Photo 9. Resisted forearm supination.   Photo 10. Resisted forearm pronation.

Next, have the patient supinate the forearm against resistance (Photo 9). This tests the patient's biceps muscle, which is innervated by the musculocutaneous nerve (C5–C6); and the supinator muscle, which is innervated by the radial nerve (C6).

Have the patient pronate the arm against resistance (Photo 10). This tests the patient's pronator teres muscle, which is innervated by the median nerve (C6); and the pronator quadratus, which is innervated by the anterior interosseous branch of the median nerve (C8–T1).

Table 1 lists the movements of the elbow, along with the involved muscles and their innervation.

Test the patient's reflexes—the biceps reflex (C5), the brachioradialis reflex (C6), and the triceps reflex (C7).

Table 1
Primary Muscles and Innervation for Elbow Movement

Major muscle movement	*Primary muscles involved*	*Primary innervation*
Elbow flexion	1. Biceps brachii and brachialis muscles.	1. Musculocutaneous nerve (C5, C6).
Elbow extension	1. Triceps.	1. Radial nerve (C7).
Forearm supination	1. Biceps.	1. Musculocutaneous nerve (C5, C6).
	2. Supinator.	2. Radial nerve (C6).
Forearm pronation	1. Pronator teres.	1. Median nerve (C6).
	2. Pronator quadratus.	2. Anterior interosseous branch of the median nerve (C8, T1).

Plan

Having completed your history and physical examination, you have a good idea of what is wrong with your patient's elbow and/or forearm. Here is what to do next:

- **Suspected lateral epicondylitis**

Additional diagnostic evaluation: Not generally necessary.
Treatment: More than 95% of patients respond well to a combination of physical therapy—including strengthening and stretching exercises—ultrasound, electrical stimulation, iontophoresis, icing, counterforce bracing (which moves the fulcrum of pressure away from the lateral epicondyle), wrist splinting, and/or steroid injections. The remaining refractory cases may be treated surgically under local anesthesia.

- **Suspected medial epicondylitis**

Additional diagnostic evaluation: Not generally necessary.
Treatment: The conservative modalities used are similar to lateral epicondylitis and are considered first-line treatment. However, conservative measures are not as successful for medial epicondylitis as they are for lateral epicondylitis. Surgery is reserved for patients with refractory symptoms.

- **Suspected ulnar collateral ligament injury**

   Additional diagnostic evaluation: X-rays, including anteroposterior (AP) and lateral views, and magnetic resonance imaging with contrast are routinely ordered.

   Treatment: Conservative care, including physical therapy, non-steroidal anti-inflammatory drugs (NSAIDs), and rest, is considered the first-line of treatment for many patients. Surgical intervention should be considered for competitive athletes hoping to return to competition and patients with symptoms that do not respond to more conservative measures.

- **Suspected fracture**

   Common fractures include humerus supracondylar fractures (most common in children), humerus intercondylar fractures (more common in adults), radial head fractures, and ulnar fractures.

   Additional diagnostic evaluation: X-rays, including AP and lateral views, should be obtained.

   Treatment: Casting and/or surgery are indicated.

- **Suspected olecranon bursitis**

   Additional diagnostic evaluation: None necessary.

   Treatment: Conservative care, including rest, activity modification, NSAIDs, and a corticosteroid and anesthetic injection into the bursa, is generally effective.

- **Suspected rheumatoid arthritis**

   Additional diagnostic evaluation: Laboratory studies including antinuclear antibody, erythrocyte sedimentation rate, rheumatoid factor, uric acid, and white blood cell levels. X-rays, including AP and lateral views, should be obtained.

   Treatment: Treating the underlying disease is important in rheumatoid arthritis. Local symptoms may be treated with rest, intra-articular corticosteroid and anesthetic injections, and physical therapy.

- **Suspected osteoarthritis**

   Additional diagnostic evaluation: X-rays, including AP and lateral views, should be obtained.

Treatment: Conservative care, including rest, physical therapy, NSAIDs, and intra-articular injection of corticosteroid and anesthetic, is appropriate treatment.

- **Suspected cubital tunnel syndrome**

Additional diagnostic evaluation: Electrodiagnostic studies are routinely obtained in order to delineate the site of nerve entrapment and the degree of nerve injury.

Treatment: Conservative care, including activity modification, splinting, and/or steroid injection, is often successful. Surgery is reserved for refractory cases.

4 Wrist and Hand Pain

First Thoughts

When your patient complains of wrist or hand pain, your differential diagnosis of most common causes is, unfortunately, a mixed bag. It includes carpal tunnel syndrome, De Quervain's tenosynovitis, ulnar collateral ligament injury (also known as "skier's thumb" or "gamekeeper's thumb"), "trigger finger," fractures, and rheumatoid arthritis. Fortunately, your history and physical examination will enable you to accurately diagnose most of these common problems.

History

Begin by asking the following questions:

1. Where is your pain?

Patients with De Quervain's tenosynovitis complain of pain over the radial styloid process. Patients with carpal tunnel syndrome complain of pain, numbness, and tingling over the wrist, palm, and the first three digits and the median half of the fourth digit. Patients with trigger finger may or may not have pain when their finger "triggers." Patients with a fracture will complain of pain over the fracture site.

2. What is the quality of your pain and/or symptoms (e.g., sharp, electric, dull, aching, numbness, tingling, etc.)?

This is another high-yield question. Patients with carpal tunnel syndrome will complain of pain, numbness, tingling, and electric sensations in their first three digits.

From: *Pocket Guide to Musculoskeletal Diagnosis*
G. Cooper

3. What are your occupation and hobbies?

Patients who work at a desk, type, or who perform other repetitive activities that involve simultaneous wrist and finger flexion are prone to develop carpal tunnel syndrome.

4. When did your symptoms begin?

This question is most useful for eliciting a history of trauma that may have precipitated a fracture. Patients with "skier's thumb" will typically describe a fall onto an outstretched arm with an abducted thumb, such as with a ski pole in their hand, preventing thumb adduction. The question also offers an indication of chronicity. More chronic symptoms are less likely to spontaneously resolve, and this information will be most helpful when deciding on what imaging studies and treatments to order.

5. Do you ever have symptoms at night that awaken you from sleep?

Night-time symptoms that wake the patient from sleep are a classic sign of carpal tunnel syndrome.

6. Have you tried any treatments for your pain and have they helped?

This question is more useful when you are deciding which diagnostic studies, if any, to order and how to treat your patient.

Physical Exam

Having completed the history portion of your examination, you have narrowed your differential diagnosis and are prepared to perform your physical exam.

Begin the physical exam by inspecting the patient's hands. Note any swelling, ecchymosis, or asymmetry. Observe the patient using their hands, noting any functional deficits. Inspect the thenar eminence and note any muscle wasting (a characteristic sign of chronic carpal tunnel syndrome). Assess the range of motion of the wrist and fingers. A sudden palpable and/or audible snapping that occurs with flexion and/or extension of one of the digits during range of motion testing is indicative of "trigger finger," which is generally caused by a fibrotic enlargement of the tendon that causes it to fail to glide smoothly through its pulley system and causes it to catch and give way as it moves in and out of the proximal sheath.

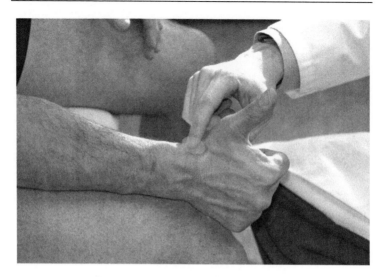

Photo 1. Anatomic snuffbox palpation.

Palpate the anatomic snuffbox, which is the small depression immediately distal and slightly dorsal to the radial styloid process (Photo 1).
Tenderness in the anatomic snuffbox suggests a scaphoid fracture. The
scaphoid bone forms the floor of the anatomic snuffbox.

Palpate the radial styloid process. Tenderness over the radial styloid
may signify De Quervain's tenosynovitis. De Quervain's tenosynovitis
is inflammation of the abductor pollicis longus and extensor pollicis
brevis tendons. To further test for De Quervain's tenosynovitis, perform the Finklestein test by instructing the patient to make a fist with
the thumb adducted and tucked inside of the other fingers. The examiner then stabilizes the forearm with one hand and deviates the wrist to
the ulnar side with the other (Photo 2). This maneuver stretches the
involved tendons. If this maneuver produces pain, the patient has a
positive Finklestein's test and may have De Quervain's tenosynovitis.

If "skier's thumb" is suspected, radiographs should be obtained to
rule out the possibility of a fracture. Once a fracture has been ruled out,
test the integrity of the ulnar collateral ligament of the first metacarpophalangeal joint. This is done by having the patient put the forearm
in the neutral position—midway between supination and pronation. The
examiner then uses a thumb and index finger to stabilize the patient's
first metacarpal. The examiner uses the thumb and index finger of the

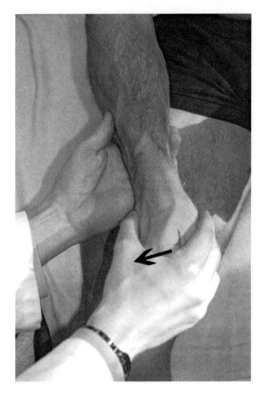

Photo 2. Finkelstein's test.

other hand to glide the patient's proximal aspect of the proximal phalanx in the radial direction until all the slack is gone. Excessive glide
reveals that the ulnar collateral ligament is injured.

Next, palpate the ulnar styloid process. Distal to the ulnar styloid
process is the tunnel of Guyon. The tunnel of Guyon is formed by
the pisiform bone, the hook of the hamate, and pisohamate ligament.
The ulnar nerve and artery run through the rigid tunnel of Guyon. The
tunnel of Guyon is a common site of ulnar nerve entrapment and injury,
potentially resulting in numbness, tingling, and weakness in the ulnar
nerve distribution of the fourth and fifth digits. If a compression neuropathy exists, the tunnel will be notably tender (Photo 3). Just proximal to the tunnel, the ulnar artery may be palpated.

Then, palpate each finger and any enlarged joints. Bouchard's nodes

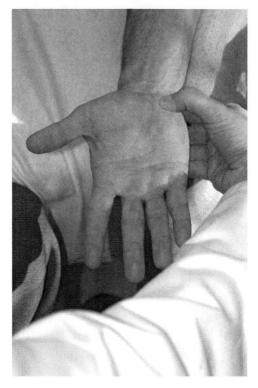

Photo 3. Tunnel of Guyon palpation.

are palpable bony nodules in the proximal interphalangeal joints and are indicative of osteoarthritis. Palpable bony nodules in the distal interphalangeal joints are called "Heberden's nodes," and are indicative of rheumatoid arthritis. Swan-neck deformity, in which the proximal interphalangeal (PIP) joint is hyperextended and the distal interphalangeal (DIP) joint is flexed, is also indicative of rheumatoid arthritis. A boutonniere deformity, in which there is hyperflexion at the PIP and hyperextension at the DIP, is also characteristic of rheumatoid arthritis.

Next, test for the integrity of the patient's flexor digitorum superficialis and flexor digitorum profundus. The flexor digitorum superficialis inserts into the middle phalanx of the finger and flexes the PIP and metacarpophalangeal joints, and the wrist. To test this muscle and tendon, maintain all but one of the patient's PIP joints in extension

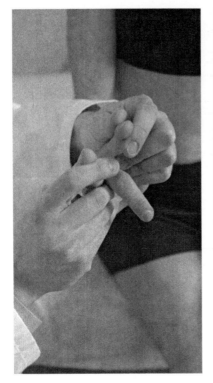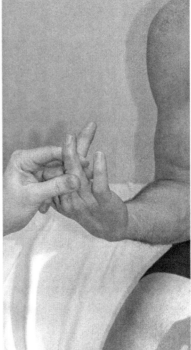

Photo 4. PIP flexion.　　　　Photo 5. DIP flexion.

and have the patient flex the remaining PIP joint (Photo 4). Next, test the patient's flexor digitorum profundus, which inserts into the distal phalanx. Note that the flexor digitorum profundus muscles to the first, second, and third digits are innervated by the median nerve. The flexor digitorum profundus muscles to the fourth and fifth digits are innervated by the ulnar nerve. To test this muscle and tendon, maintain the patient's PIP joint in extension and have the patient flex each individual DIP joint (Photo 5).

The median nerve passes through the carpal tunnel, which is a rigid tunnel surrounded on three sides by wrist bones and anteriorly by the dense transverse carpal ligament. Because of its rigidity, any increase in carpal tunnel pressure may result in compression of the median

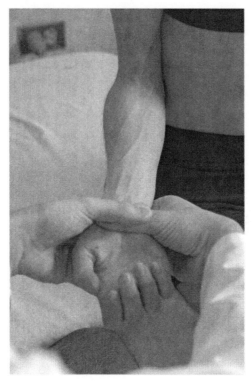

Photo 6. Compression test.

nerve, resulting in paresthesias in the first, second, and third digits and the median half of the fourth digit. Three clinical examination tools are used to assess for carpal tunnel syndrome. First, tap repetitively over the median nerve as it passes through the carpal tunnel. This is Tinel's test for carpal tunnel syndrome and it is positive when the tapping reproduces your patient's symptoms in the first three digits (Tinel's test is the most specific clinical test for carpal tunnel syndrome). Next, perform the compression test, which is the most sensitive test for carpal tunnel syndrome. To perform this test, apply continuous pressure over the patient's carpal tunnel for 60 seconds (Photo 6). If this maneuver reproduces the patient's symptoms, the test is positive. Finally, perform Phalen's test. To perform this test, instruct the patient to hold both of the wrists in flexion against one another for 60 seconds (Photo 7). This test is positive if the position reproduces the patient's symptoms.

Next, test the patient's strength. Have the patient extend the wrist against resistance (Photo 8). This tests the extensor carpi radialis longus, extensor carpi radialis brevis, and extensor carpi ulnaris mus-

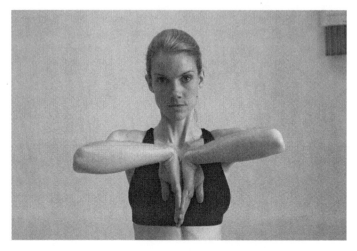

Photo 7. Phalen's test.

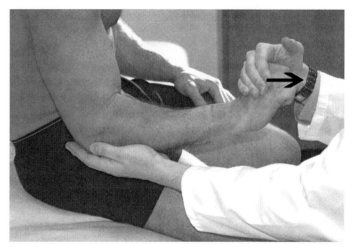

Photo 8. Resisted wrist flexion.

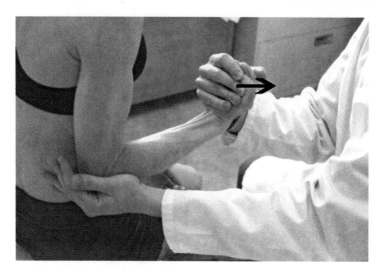

Photo 9. Resisted wrist flexion.

cles, which are all innervated by the radial nerve (predominately C6).

Have the patient flex the wrist against resistance (Photo 9). This tests the patient's flexor carpi radialis muscle, which is innervated by the median nerve (C7); and the flexor carpi ulnaris muscle, which is innervated by the ulnar nerve (C8–T1). Despite the multiple nerve involvement, wrist flexion is predominately mediated by C7.

Next, have the patient flex their fingers against resistance. Finger flexion is predominately mediated by C8.

Then have the patient abduct and adduct their fingers against resistance. This is predominately mediated by T1.

Test the integrity of the patient's anterior interosseous nerve by having the patient make the "OK" sign (Photo 10). If the patient has an anterior interosseous neuropathy, the patient will be unable to make the "OK" sign (Photo 11).

Table 1 lists the major movements of the hand and wrist, along with the involved muscles and their innervation.

Finally, test for sensory deficits (Photo 12). The C6 dermatome is tested over the dorsal aspect of the first proximal phalanx; the C7 dermatome is tested over the dorsal aspect of the third proximal phalanx; and the C8 dermatome is tested over the dorsal aspect of the fifth proximal phalanx. Test for the radial nerve sensory distribution in the

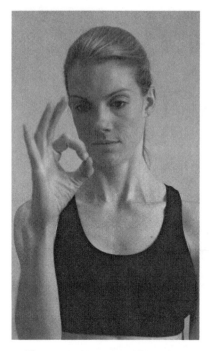

Photo 10. Negative "OK" sign.

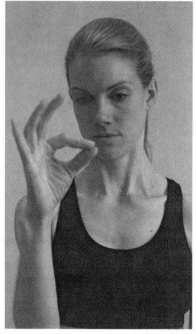

Photo 11. Simulated positive "OK" sign in anterior interosseous nerve lesion.

web space between the first and second fingers.

Plan

Having completed your history and physical examination, you have a good idea of what is wrong with your patient's wrist and hand. Here is what to do next:

- **Suspected carpal tunnel syndrome**

Additional diagnostic evaluation: Electrodiagnostic studies should be performed if the diagnosis is in doubt or if surgery is considered.

Treatment: Conservative care, including activity modification and splinting in the neutral position, are the cornerstones of first-line treatment. Tendon gliding exercises and corticosteroid and anesthetic injec-

Table 1
Primary Muscles and Innervation for Wrist and Finger Movement

Major muscle movement	Primary muscles involved	Primary nerve innervation
Wrist extension	1. Extensor carpi radialis longus, extensor carpi radialis brevis, and extensor carpi ulnaris.	1. Radial nerve (predominately C6).
Wrist flexion	1. Flexor carpi radialis. 2. Flexor carpi ulnaris.	1. Median nerve (C7). 2. Ulnar nerve (C8, T1). **Note:** the primary innervation of wrist flexion is from C7.
Finger flexion	1. Flexor digitorum superficialis and flexor digitorum profundus.	1. Median and ulnar nerves. **Note:** finger flexion is predominately C8.
Finger abduction and adduction	1. Dorsal interossei abduct and the palmar interossei adduct.	1. Ulnar nerve. **Note:** finger abduction and adduction is predominately T1.

tions may also be helpful. In patients with refractory symptoms, surgical release is very effective.

• **Suspected De Quervain's tenosynovitis**

Additional diagnostic evaluation: None necessary.

Treatment: Often the only treatment necessary is reassurance and avoidance of the offending activity. Splinting may be used. Corticosteroid injections into the sheath are also helpful. Caution must be exercised with corticosteroid injections because subcutaneous injections may result in skin hypopigmentation. After one or two corticosteroid and anesthetic injections into the sheath, 90 to 95% of patients report sat-

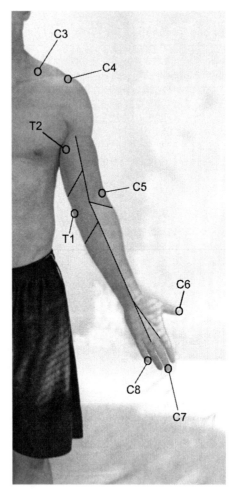

Photo 12. Upper dermatome with circles indicating location to test. (Note that C6–C8 should be on the dorsal surface.

isfactory results. Surgery is reserved for refractory cases.

- **Suspected rheumatoid arthritis**

Additional diagnostic evaluation: Laboratory studies including antinuclear antibody, erythrocyte sedimentation rate, rheumatoid factor, uric acid, and white blood cell levels. X-rays, including anteroposterior (AP) and lateral views, should be obtained.

Treatment: Treating the underlying rheumatoid arthritis is important. Further treatment includes splinting the involved joints and rest. Surgery may also be necessary.

- **Suspected osteoarthritis**

Additional diagnostic evaluation: X-rays, including AP and lateral views, should be obtained.

Treatment: Acetaminophen, nonsteroidal anti-inflammatory drugs (NSAIDs), steroid injections, heat, and physical therapy are all first-line treatments.

- **Suspected trigger finger**

Additional diagnostic evaluation: None necessary.

Treatment: A combination of splinting and corticosteroid and anesthetic injections is effective in more than 95% of patients. The remaining patients with refractory symptoms may require surgery.

- **Suspected anterior interosseous nerve syndrome**

Additional diagnostic evaluation: X-rays, including AP and lateral views, may be obtained to rule out more serious underlying pathology.

Treatment: First-line treatment includes rest, NSAIDs, splinting, and physical therapy. Surgical release may be necessary in patients who do not respond to more conservative measures.

- **Suspected ganglion cyst**

Additional diagnostic evaluation: X-rays, including AP and lateral views, may be obtained to rule out more serious underlying pathology.

Treatment: If the ganglion cyst is asymptomatic, then simple reassurance may be all that is necessary. If the cyst becomes symptomatic or if it is aesthetically unacceptable to the patient, aspiration or surgical excision may be performed. Aspiration has a higher recurrent rate than excision.

- **Suspected fracture**

Common fractures include radial head fracture, olecranon fracture, Greenstick fracture, scaphoid fracture, lunate fracture, metacarpal fracture (most commonly the fifth metacarpal—Boxer's fracture), and phalanx fracture (most commonly the fifth phalanx).

Additional diagnostic evaluation: X-rays, including AP, lateral, ulnar deviation, and oblique views (depending on the fracture suspected), should be obtained. Computed tomography and/or magnetic resonance imaging are also often necessary.

Treatment: Splinting and/or surgery.

Special consideration: Patients with snuffbox tenderness but negative radiographs should be treated with 2 weeks of a thumb spica followed by repeat X-rays to rule out scaphoid fracture because of the risk of avascular necrosis. Fractures are generally treated with casting and/or surgery.

5   Low Back, Hip, and Shooting Leg Pain

First Thoughts, Basic (and a Little Not-So-Basic) Pathophysiology

Because the underlying pathologies of low back, hip, and shooting leg pain (radicular pain) reside within the low back and/or hip, essentially the same physical examination is performed for each complaint. Therefore, all three complaints are discussed in this chapter. As in the cervical spine, because the diagnostic and therapeutic approach to radicular and nociceptive pain is very different, it is important to distinguish them during the history and physical examination. Understanding the language of low back pain is as important as understanding the language of neck pain. You may wish to briefly review the principles and terminologies discussed at the beginning of Chapter 1.

In the lumbosacral spine, radicular symptoms are caused by an intervertebral disc bulge, protrusion, extrusion, or sequestration that compresses and inflames a nerve root in approximately 98% of all cases. Other causes of radicular symptoms emanating from the lumbosacral spine include disc osteophytes, a buckled ligamentum flavum, zygapophysial (Z)-joint hypertrophy, and other causes of lumbosacral spinal stenosis.

Axial low back pain is defined as "pain perceived within a region bounded superiorly by a transverse line through the T12 spinous process, laterally by the lateral borders of erector spinae muscles and posterior superior iliac spinous processes, and inferiorly by a transverse line through sacrococcygial joints." In the low back, referral pain patterns commonly present in the hip or leg. A classic example of a referral pain pattern in the lumbosacral spine is low back pain associated with aching buttock pain. The lumbosacral region and buttocks are both innervated by L4–S1. However, the buttock is innervated by the ventral rami of

From: *Pocket Guide to Musculoskeletal Diagnosis*
G. Cooper

these nerve roots (the superior and inferior gluteal nerves), and the lumbosacral region is innervated by the dorsal rami. The brain is sometimes unable to distinguish whether axial low back pain is actually originating from the buttocks or low back (because both fibers use the L4–S1 nerve roots). Low back pain is therefore sometimes perceived in a poorly defined distribution in *both* the low back and buttocks.

Acute low back pain lasts less than 3 months. Numerous potential causes of low back pain, including more vague diagnoses, such as "muscle strain," "muscle tightness," and "myofascial pain," have been reported. Evidence to support these assertions is often limited and anecdotal. Conventional wisdom has been that 90% of cases of acute low back pain spontaneously resolve. The true story is somewhat more complicated. In fact, systematic evaluation of the data has revealed that anywhere from 40 to 90% of acute low back pain may initially resolve prior to 3 months. A more common picture of low back pain may be one of periodic remissions and relapses.

However, when low back pain becomes chronic (lasting more than 3 months), the evidence regarding its etiology and pathophysiology is much more scientific and complete. In fact, research has shown that there are three common causes of chronic low back pain. Each of these causes has been scientifically validated and each is readily identified when the proper diagnostic investigations are rigorously pursued.

Chronic low back pain has been shown to be caused by a painful intervertebral disc (discogenic low back pain) in approximately 39% of cases, a diseased Z-joint in up to 30% of cases, and sacroiliac joint disease in approximately 15% of cases.

History

Ask the patient the following questions:

1. Where is your pain?

This question will help you distinguish nociceptive pain from radicular pain (hip pain and axial low back pain are both nociceptive pain and must ultimately be distinguished during the physical examination). Hip pain is often perceived in the hip and/or groin, although it may also be perceived in the knee. Common causes of hip pain include dislocation, fracture, and osteoarthritis. Axial low back pain with a referral pain pattern may also occur in the hip. It is more common, however, for axial low back pain with referral pain to occur in the buttocks and/or leg(s) in a pattern that is difficult to

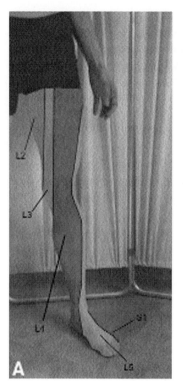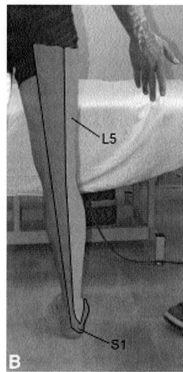

Photo 1. Lower extremity dermatome patterns. (A) Anterior, (B) posterior.

localize. Radicular pain, by contrast, is band-like and more easily localized as it radiates down the leg. Radicular symptoms over the anterior thigh that end at the knee are typically associated with the L3 nerve root. Radicular symptoms that extend over the medial knee, medial calf, and medial malleolus are typically associated with the L4 nerve root. Radicular symptoms that occur over the dorsum of the foot are typically associated with L5. Radicular symptoms that occur along the back of the thigh and the lateral heel are typically associated with S1. It is rare to have radicular symptoms from S2 or below. Photo 1 demonstrates the characteristic dermatomes of the lower extremity (Photo 1). Although knowing the location and distribution of pain is helpful, further questioning is necessary to determine if the pain is truly radicular, axial low back (with or without a referral pattern), or hip pain.

2. **What is the quality of your pain (e.g., shooting, electric, dull, aching, etc.)?**

   This is the question that will definitively tell you if the patient has radicular pain or axial pain. Radicular pain is sharp, shooting, and electric. Nociceptive pain (axial low back and hip pain) and referred pain are *not* sharp, shooting, or electric. This is an easy, and very important, distinction to make.

3. **How long have you had pain?**

   This is a particularly important question for low back pain. Acute low back pain is defined as low back pain lasting less than 3 months and is much more likely to spontaneously resolve than chronic low back pain. Therefore, aggressive diagnosis and treatment of acute low back pain may not be necessary.

4. **Do any positions aggravate or relieve your symptoms?**

   Patients with radicular symptoms caused by spinal stenosis will classically complain of pain aggravated by leaning backward. These patients also have improved symptoms with trunk flexion. This is often referred to as the "shopping cart sign." In this sign, the patient reports improvement of symptoms while shopping because the patient leans forward while pushing the shopping cart. By contrast, patients with a disc herniation causing radicular symptoms will report *increased* symptoms with trunk flexion. This is because trunk flexion increases the intradiscal pressure.

5. **Have you tried anything to help your pain?**

   This question is most useful for when you are deciding which diagnostic studies to order, if any, and for selecting treatment options.

6. **Have you experienced any recent night sweats, weight loss, hematuria, urinary retention, frequency, hesitancy, or cough? Do you have a history of cancer, overseas travel, recent surgery, fever, or increased pain at rest? Has your pain ever woken you from sleep?**

   These questions should be asked of every patient with low back, hip, or radicular symptoms in order to help screen more serious underlying conditions such as a tumor or infection.

7. **Have you had any recent change in bowel or bladder habits? Do you have any altered sensation in your groin, buttocks, or inner thighs?**

   These questions should be asked of every patient with suspected spinal pathology to help rule out cord impingement, conus medullaris, and cauda equina syndrome.

Physical Exam

Having completed the history portion of your examination, you have distinguished whether or not your patient has nociceptive pain (remember that low back and hip pain must be distinguished during the physical examination) or radicular pain. You have also begun to narrow your differential diagnosis. It is now time to perform your physical exam.

Begin by observing the patient's gait. Is the gait antalgic (i.e., does the patient limp or favor one leg over the other)? Instruct the patient to stand on one foot and then the other. This is the Trendelenberg test, and it is performed to examine the integrity of the gluteus medius muscle. If one gluteus medius muscle is weak, when the patient stands on the weak side, the patient's pelvis will shift upwards to the ipsilateral side of weakness and the patient's trunk will lurch to the contralateral side in order to maintain the patient's center of gravity (Photo 2).

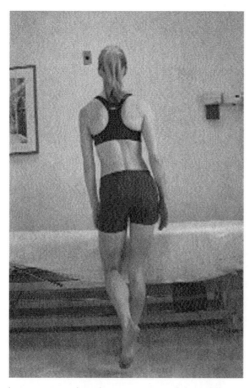

Photo 2. Simulated positive Trendelenberg sign.

Standing behind the patient, observe for any apparent leg length discrepancy (the true leg length may be measured from the anterior superior iliac spine to the medial malleolus; however, using a tape measure is not generally necessary unless leg length discrepancy is suspected on general observation).

Palpate the vertebral bodies. Tenderness over the vertebral bodies should prompt further investigation for a vertebral metastasis or compression fracture. Palpate the paraspinal muscles for any muscle spasms, tender points, or trigger points (**Note:** trigger points are defined as discrete areas of tenderness that also have a referral pain pattern when palpated; tender points are tender but have *no* referral pain pattern). Palpate the soft tissues over the posterior portion of the greater trochanter (Photo 3). Tenderness in this region may indicate trochanteric bursitis.

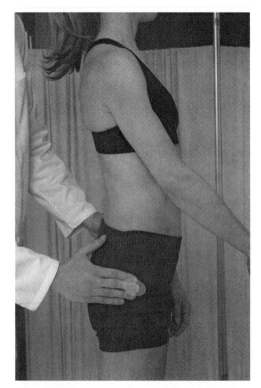

Photo 3. Greater trochanter bursa palpation.

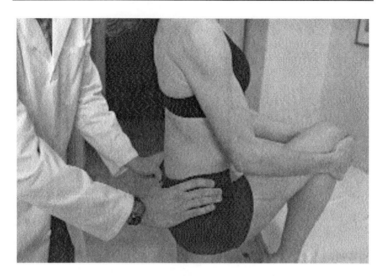

Photo 4. Gillet's test.

Remain standing behind the patient and place one thumb on the posterior superior iliac spine and the other thumb on the patient's sacrum. Instruct the patient to stand on one leg and have the patient pull the opposite leg to the chest (Photo 4). This is Gillet's test, and it is used to test for sacroiliac joint involvement. In a patient with a normal sacroiliac joint, the ipsilateral posterior superior iliac spine should move inferiorly. If the posterior superior iliac spine is felt to move superiorly, then the joint is described as hypomobile, and may be contributing to the patient's pain. Repeat the test in the opposite leg.

Next, instruct the patient to bend over as far as the patient can comfortably go. Observe the patient's spine for any asymmetry or scoliosis. Trunk flexion increases intradiscal pressures. If bending over reproduces shooting leg pain or other radicular symptoms (e.g., numbness or tingling), the patient may have a herniated disc.

Next, instruct the patient to lean backwards as far as is comfortable. Then, obliquely extend the patient's spine first to the right, and then to the left (Photo 5). This maneuver stresses the posterior elements of the spine. If extension or oblique extension reproduces the patient's low back pain, the patient may have Z-joint pain. If extension or oblique extension reproduces shooting leg pain or other radicular symptoms, the patient may have foraminal stenosis.

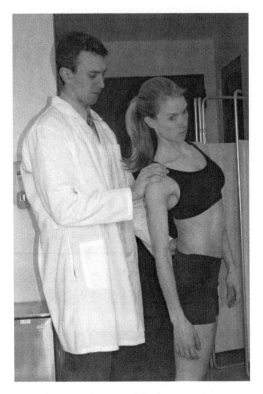

Photo 5. Passive obique extension.

Ask the patient to stand on one leg and extend backward toward the supporting leg (Photo 6). Repeat the test with the patient standing on the other leg. This is the Stork Standing test, and if pain is reproduced with the test, the patient may have a pars interarticularis stress fracture (spondylolisthesis). If the stress fracture is unilateral, standing on the ipsilateral leg and bending backwards toward that leg will be most painful.

Next, have the patient sit down. Instruct the patient to lean forward and touch the chin to the chest. Then, slowly extend the leg (Photo 7). This is a dural tension test. If this reproduces radicular symptoms radiating down the patient's leg, the patient may have nerve root compression and/or inflammation.

With the patient still seated, internally and externally rotate the patient's hip using the ankle as a lever (Photos 8 and 9). If this maneuver

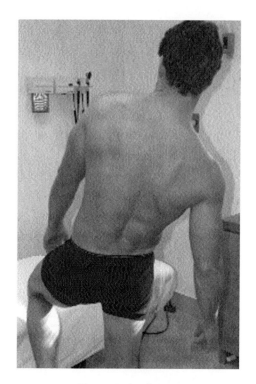

Photo 6. Stork test.

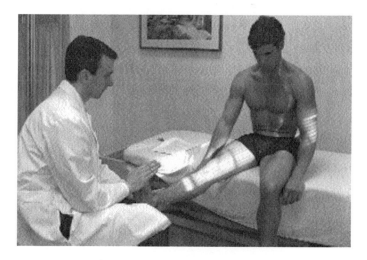

Photo 7. Seated dural tension sign.

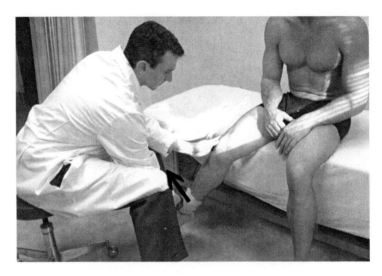

Photo 8. Hip internal rotation.

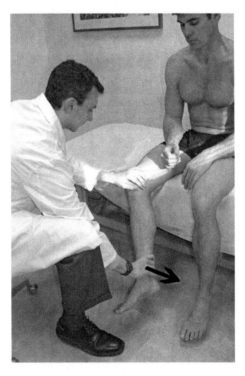

Photo 9. Hip external rotation.

reproduces the patient's pain, the patient's hip (or even back) pain may be originating from the hip. If this does not reproduce the patient's pain, the patient probably does not have hip pathology causing the pain.

Next, have the patient flex the hip against resistance (Photo 10). This tests the patient's iliopsoas muscle, which is innervated by the femoral nerve (L1–L3).

Have the patient extend the knee against resistance (Photo 11). This tests the patient's quadriceps, which are innervated by the femoral nerve (L2–L4).

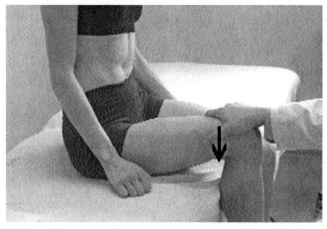

Photo 10. Hip flexion against resistance.

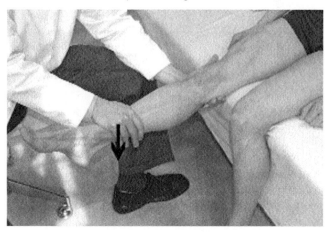

Photo 11. Knee extension against resistance.

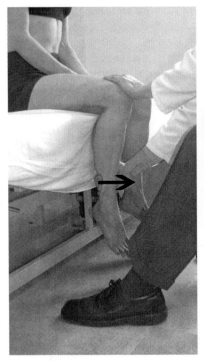 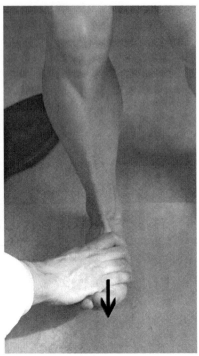

Photo 12. Knee flexion against   Photo 13. Ankle dorsiflexion against
resistance.   resistance.

Next, have the patient flex the knee against resistance (Photo 12).
This tests the patient's hamstrings, which are innervated primarily by
the tibial portion of the sciatic nerve (L5, S1; the short head of the
biceps femoris is innervated by the common peroneal division of the
sciatic nerve, L5–S2).

With the patient's heel planted on the ground, instruct them to dorsiflex the ankle against resistance (Photo 13). This tests the patient's
tibialis anterior, which is innervated by the deep peroneal nerve
(L4, L5).

Next, have the patient plantarflex against resistance (Photo 14).
This tests the patient's gastrocnemius and soleus muscles, which are
innervated by the tibial nerve (S1).

Have the patient extend the big toe against resistance (Photo 15).
This is an important test because the big toe (hallucis longus) is

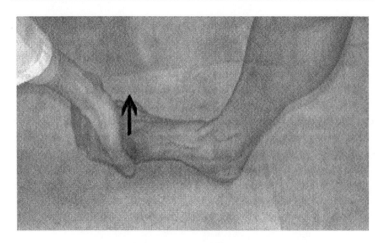

Photo 14. Ankle plantar flexion against resistance.

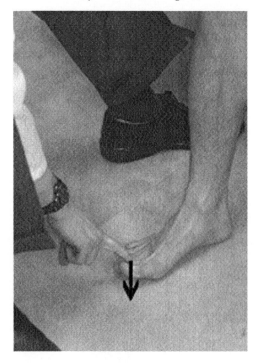

Photo 15. Big toe extension against resistance.

extended by the extensor hallucis longus, which is innervated almost exclusively by the L5 nerve root. In a patient with a suspected radiculopathy, extensor hallucis longus weakness is a specific clinical indicator for involvement of the L5 nerve root.

With the patient still seated, it is convenient to test the reflexes. Test the patella reflex (L4) and the Achilles reflex (S1) (Photos 16 and 17). Test for an upper motor neuron deficit by evaluating for a Babinski reflex. To evaluate for this reflex, the examiner runs a sharp instrument along the plantar surface of the foot, starting at the calcaneus and moving along the lateral border and then curving around to the big toe (Photo 18). The patient has a Babinski reflex if the patient extends the big toe and flexes the rest of the toes. If the patient flexes the big toe or if there is no reaction, then there is no Babisnki reflex. In patients without an upper motor neuron lesion, the Babinski reflex disappears around the first year of life. The presence of a Babinski reflex therefore indicates an upper motor neuron lesion.

It is now appropriate to perform a quick test of sensation (Photo 19). The L3 dermatome is tested over the medial femoral condyle; the L4 dermatome is tested over the medial malleolus; the L5 dermatome is tested over the dorsal aspect of the third or fifth digit; and the S1 der-

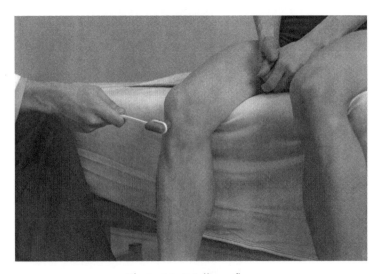

Photo 16. Patellar reflex.

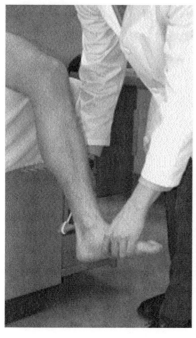

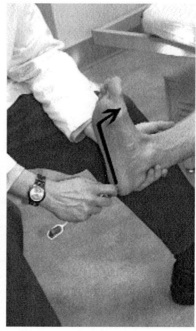

Photo 17. Achilles reflex.   Photo 18. Babinski reflex elicitation.

matome is tested over the lateral aspect of the heel. Compare both sides of the body for symmetry and note any numbness or dysethesias.

Finally, with the patient still seated, check for pulses behind the knees in the popliteal arteries bilaterally and the posterior tibial arteries behind the medial malleolus bilaterally.

Now have the patient lie in the supine position. Instruct the patient to adduct the hips against resistance (Photo 20). This tests the patient's adductor longus muscle, which is innervated by the obturator nerve (L2–L4).

The Hoover test is helpful in identifying potential malingering patients. With the patient supine, cup your hands underneath both of the patient's heels. Instruct the patient to lift one heel off the table. When the patient is truly attempting to lift the leg off the table, he or she will automatically put downward pressure on the opposite heel (which you will feel in your palm). If the patient states that pain prevents them from

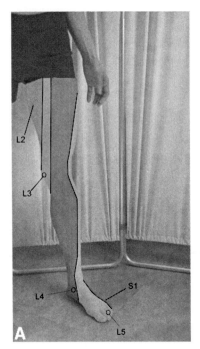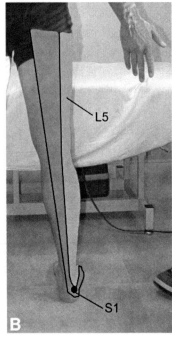

Photo 19. Lower extremity dermatomes with dots indicate where to test for sensation. (A) Anterior, (B) posterior.

raising the leg, but you do not feel downward pressure in the contralateral palm, the patient is probably not really attempting to raise the leg.

Next, take the patient's extended leg and slowly raise it (flexing the patient's hip; Photo 21). This is the straight leg-raise test. If this maneuver reproduces the patient's radicular symptoms shooting down the leg, the patient may have a pathological process (most commonly a disc protrusion) compressing and inflaming the nerve root. Typically, the maneuver reproduces radicular symptoms at 35–70° of hip flexion. It is at this amount of flexion that the nerves are maximally stretched. If the patient complains of pain but is unclear if the pain is radicular in nature, dorsiflex the ankle. If ankle dorsiflexion does not increase the symptoms, then the symptoms are more likely to be the result of hamstring tightness. If radicular symptoms are "reproduced" after 70° of flexion, the result is more likely to be a false positive.

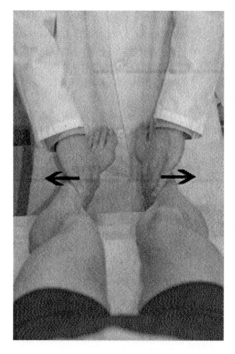

Photo 20. Hip adduction against resistance.

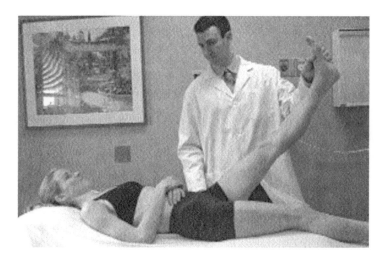

Photo 21. Straight leg raise.

Now take hold of the patient's knee and ankle, and with the hip and knee flexed to approximately 90°, move the hip into internal and then external rotation. This is a convenient and effective way to test for hip pathology again. If this maneuver reproduces the patient's pain, the hip may be the underlying cause of the symptoms. If this fails to reproduce the patient's pain, the hip is unlikely to be involved.

With the patient still lying in the supine position, perform the Thomas test to assess for tight hip flexors. To perform the Thomas test, have the patient lie in the supine position and flex one hip so that the patient is hugging one knee to the chest. If the patient has a tight hip

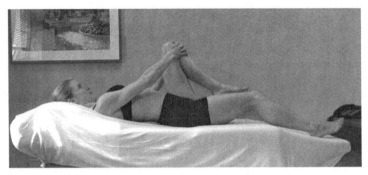

Photo 22. Simulated positive Thomas test.

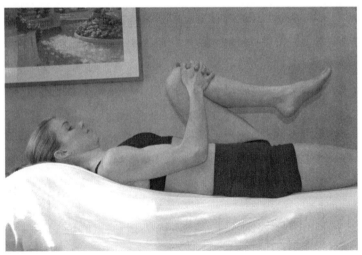

Photo 23. Negative Thomas test.

flexor, the extended leg (the leg being tested) will lift off the table (Photo 22). If the patient does not have a tight hip flexor, the extended leg will remain flat on the table when the patient hugs the other knee to the chest (Photo 23).

Next, test for a sacroiliac joint or hip injury by performing the Faber test. Faber is an acronym for flexion, abduction, and external rotation. To perform this test (the patient should be supine), place the foot of the involved side onto the opposite knee in a "figure-4" position (thus flexing, abducting, and externally rotating the affected hip. If this produces pain in the inguinal region, the hip joint may be involved. Further stress the sacroiliac joint by pushing down on the flexed knee, as well as on the contralateral superior iliac spine. If this maneuver produces pain, the sacroiliac joint may be involved.

Next, have the patient lie on his or her side. Instruct the patient to abduct the hip against resistance (Photo 24). This tests the patient's gluteus medius, which is innervated by the superior gluteal nerve (primarily L5).

Next, with the patient still lying on his or her side, test for a tight iliotibial band by performing Ober's test. In this test, flex the patient's hip and knee that are lying on the table (this is done for stability). Then, take the patient's other leg (the one not in contact with the table) and

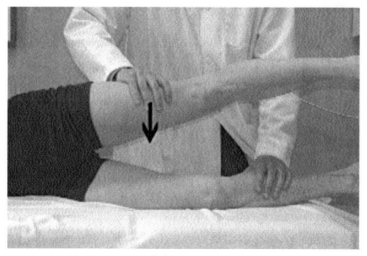

Photo 24. Hip abduction against resistance.

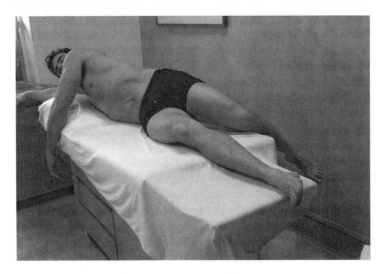

Photo 25. Negative Ober test.

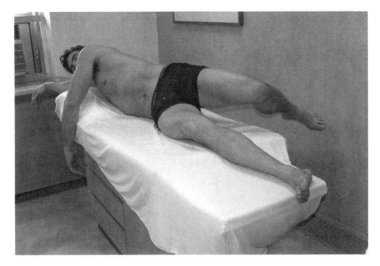

Photo 26. Simulated positive Ober test.

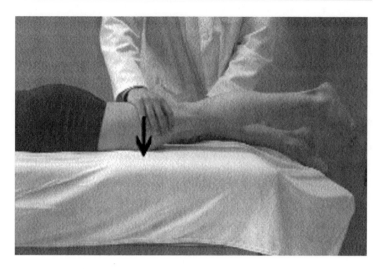

Photo 27. Hip extension against resistance.

passively abduct and extend the hip with the knee flexed to 90°. Next, slowly allow the upper leg to fall to the table. If the iliotibial band is not tight, the leg will fall to the table (Photo 25). If the iliotibial band is tight, the upper leg will not fall to the table but instead, will remain in the air (Photo 26). This test also places stress on the femoral nerve, and if it invokes paresthesias in the leg, femoral nerve pathology should be considered. If the test is performed with the knee extended, less stress is placed on the femoral nerve. Have the patient roll onto the other side and repeat testing of the hip abductor and Ober's test.

Have the patient lie in the prone position and instruct the patient to extend the hip against resistance (Photo 27). This tests the gluteus maximus, which is innervated by the inferior gluteal nerve (S1).

Table 1 lists the major movements of the hip and leg, along with the involved muscles and their innervation.

Next, test for a tight rectus femoris by performing Ely's test. In this test, passively flex your patient's knee (Photo 28). If the patient's ipsilateral hip spontaneously flexes, this is an indication that the rectus femoris is tight (Photo 29).

With your patient still in the prone position, passively extend the hip and flex the knee. If this maneuver reproduces shooting leg pain, there may be a radiculopathy involving L2–L4.

Table 1
Primary Muscles and Innervation
for Hip, Knee, Ankle, and Big Toe Movement

Major muscle movement	Primary muscle(s) involved	Primary innervation
Hip flexion	Iliopsoas.	Femoral nerve (primarily L3).
Hip extension	Gluteus maximus.	Inferior gluteal nerve (primarily S1).
Hip adduction	Adductor longus.	Obturator nerve (L2–L4).
Hip abduction	Gluteus medius and gluteus minimus.	Superior gluteal nerve (primarily L5).
Knee flexion	Hamstrings (semimembranosus, semitendinosus, biceps femoris).	Primarily tibial but also peroneal portion of sciatic nerve (primarily L5).
Knee extension	Quadriceps (vastus lateralis, vastus medialis, vastus intermedius, rectus femoris).	Femoral nerve (primarily L4).
Ankle dorsiflexion	Tibialis anterior.	Deep peroneal nerve (primarily L4).
Ankle plantarflexion	Gastrocnemius, soleus.	Tibial nerve (primarily S1).
Big toe extension	Extensor hallucis longus.	Deep peroneal nerve (primarily L5).

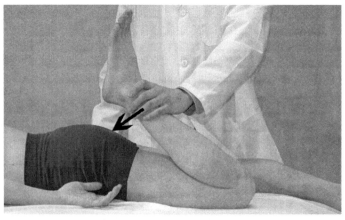

Photo 28. Negative Ely's test.

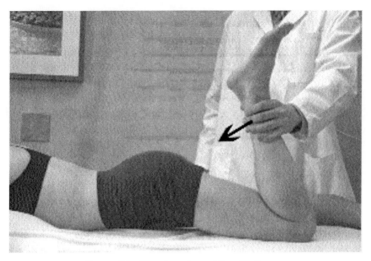

Photo 29. Simulated positive Ely's test.

Plan

Having completed your history and physical examination, you have a good idea of what is causing your patient's symptoms. Here is what to do next:

- **Suspected lumbosacral radiculopathy**

Additional diagnostic evaluation: X-rays, including anteroposterior (AP) and lateral views, are indicated. Magnetic resonance imaging (MRI) is also indicated. Electrodiagnostic studies may be used to better localize the exact lesion and evaluate for a potential peripheral neuropathy.

Treatment: Conservative treatment, including physical therapy, nonsteroidal anti-inflammatory drugs (NSAIDs), and fluoroscopically guided epidural steroid injections, have shown good efficacy for treating most radiculopathies. Surgery is reserved for refractory cases or cases with progressive neurological deficiencies (i.e., bowel or bladder changes).

- **Suspected acute low back pain**

Additional diagnostic evaluation: Unless a more serious underlying cause is suspected (e.g., fracture, tumor), no imaging is necessary.

Treatment: Physical therapy, ergonomic training, heat, activity modification, and NSAIDs may be used as first-line therapy. Instructions on good back hygiene, including sleeping with a pillow beneath the knees when supine and using a pillow between the knees when sleeping on the side, should also be offered. If any specific muscle tightness was identified during the exam, special attention should be paid to stretching for those muscles. If trigger points are identified, trigger point injections of a local anesthetic and normal saline with or without corticosteroids may be helpful.

- **Suspected chronic low back pain**

Chronic low back pain is a diagnosis that deserves special mention. The physical exam may suggest a particular cause for chronic low back pain, but the physical exam will *not* be able to offer a conclusive diagnosis in the majority of cases of chronic low back pain. To diagnose most cases, it is necessary to perform a needle procedure. For example, in order to diagnose discogenic chronic low back pain (which accounts for approximately 39% of all chronic low back pain), it is necessary to perform a discogram (a needle procedure in which dye is injected into the intervertebral disc). In order to diagnose sacroiliac joint disease (which accounts for approximately 15% of all chronic low back pain), it is necessary to anesthetize the sacroiliac joint. In order to diagnose chronic low back pain caused by Z-joint disease (which accounts for approximately 30% of chronic low back pain), it is necessary to perform controlled blocks of the nerves innervating the putative joint(s). All of these diagnostic procedures are routinely done by an orthopedist, interventional physiatrist, or pain medicine specialist. Your history, physical exam, and radiographic findings are important in helping to guide your decision of which needle procedure to perform first.

Additional diagnostic evaluation: Needle procedures should be performed as mentioned. X-rays, including AP and lateral views, are indicated. Oblique X-ray should be obtained if a pars interarticularlis fracture is suspected. MRI is also indicated.

Treatment: Conservative care similar to that for acute low back pain may be tried if the patient has not previously had a trial of conservative modalities. If a discogram reveals that the disc is the source of pain, intradiscal electrothermal annuloplasty is a minimally invasive needle procedure that has been shown to help more than half of all patients. Surgical options, including fusion surgery, are also available.

If controlled blocks reveal the Z-joint to be the source of pain, radiofrequency neurotomy is an effective needle procedure for denervating the joints and relieving the pain.

- **Suspected spondylolysis**

Additional diagnostic evaluation: AP-, lateral-, and oblique-view X-rays (**Note:** an oblique lumbar view is necessary in this instance, but also note that oblique views require significantly more radiation when compared with AP and lateral views and so should be obtained only when indicated). Computed tomography (CT) may also be necessary, particularly if the lesion is suspected (e.g., young gymnast with low back pain that is worse with activity and worse with lumbar extension) but not seen on X-ray.

Treatment: Physical therapy with emphasis on posture and body biomechanics training is instituted. Activity modification is also important. Bracing may be used. Surgery should generally be considered only in those patients who have failed conservative care. If surgical fusion of the lesion is considered, a successful diagnostic block of the pars defect is a good predictor of a successful response to fusion.

- **Suspected trochanteric bursitis**

Additional diagnostic evaluation: X-rays, including AP and lateral views, may be used to rule out a fracture or bony lesion.

Treatment: Ice, NSAIDs, heat, and physical therapy with emphasis placed on stretching the iliotibial band, hip flexors, and hip extensors may be used. A trochanteric bursa injection of anesthetic and corticosteroid injection should be considered.

- **Suspected hip osteoarthritis**

Additional diagnostic evaluation: X-rays, including AP and lateral views, are indicated.

Treatment: Treatment is based on degree of morbidity. The cornerstone of conservative care includes reducing stressful activities, resting, weight reduction (when appropriate), using ambulatory aides (e.g., cane), heat modalities, and physical therapy, including nonimpact exercises (e.g., swimming). Oral glucosamine sulfate (1500 mg) and chondroitin sulfate (1200 mg) are useful when taken daily. Intra-articular injections of anesthetic and corticosteroid may also be helpful.

The decision to treat surgically is largely guided by the patient's comorbidities, expectations, and degree of symptoms. The most common surgery for hip osteoarthritis is total hip replacement.

• Suspected hip fracture

More common hip fractures include femoral neck fractures, intertrochanteric fractures, and subtrochanteric fractures. Acetabular fractures are less common and typically require a high energy trauma.

Additional diagnostic evaluation: X-rays, including AP and lateral views, are indicated. CT and/or MRI are also generally indicated.

Treatment: Surgery is indicated, and the sooner the fracture is reduced, the better.

• Suspected hip dislocation

Additional diagnostic evaluation: X-rays, including AP and lateral views are indicated. CT and/or MRI are also indicated.

Treatment: Surgery is indicated, and the sooner the hip is reduced, the better.

6 Knee Pain

First Thoughts

When your patient complains of "knee pain," without hearing another word, your differential diagnosis includes four basic etiologies:

1. Osteoarthritis.
2. Ligament damage.
3. Meniscus damage.
4. Patellofemoral disorder.

Pes anserinus bursitis, Osgood-Schlatter disease, osteochondritis dissecans, and fractures are among the other less likely causes you will need to consider. A basic history will help you narrow the diagnosis.

History

Ask the following questions:

1. Where is your pain?

This is a very high-yield question. Have your patient point to the most painful point, if possible. Pain at the joint line is the result of a collateral ligament or meniscus problem (or both) until proven otherwise. Pain at the tibial tuberosity in a young patient is Osgood-Schlatter's syndrome until proven otherwise; anterior knee pain may be a patellofemoral disorder; pain over the medial tibial plateau, approximately 2 inches below the joint line, may be pes anserinus bursitis; and pain and swelling in the posterior knee may be a Baker's cyst.

2. When did your pain begin, what were you doing at the time, and what were the initial symptoms?

This is another high-yield question. In fact, having already ascertained the location of pain, knowing the mechanism of injury and initial symptoms will give you the diagnosis in more than half of all cases of knee pain. If the patient has a ligament injury, the patient will report a deceleration injury or twisting the knee that led to immediate symptoms of swelling and pain. In fact, 30 to 50% of patients will report actually hearing a "pop" at the time of injury. In contrast, patients with meniscus injuries may have a similar mechanism of injury (twisting or deceleration), but the patient will not notice swelling (if swelling occurs at all) until minutes or hours after the injury. There is also no "popping" sensation or sound in meniscus injuries. In an older patient, a meniscus injury may be more insidious and the patient may not recall an inciting traumatic event. Likewise, patients with osteoarthritis, patellofemoral syndrome, and Osgood-Schlatter's syndrome have a more chronic onset of symptoms. Patients with fractures will generally report a history of trauma.

3. **Do you experience any grinding, locking, catching, or giving way of the knee?**

This question is the last general high-yield question for most cases of knee pain. Grinding is characteristic of osteoarthritis; locking and catching are characteristic of meniscus injuries and osteochondritis dissecans (meniscus injuries are much more common than osteochondritis dissecans); and giving way is more characteristic of ligamentous injuries.

4. **Are there any positions that make your knee more or less comfortable?**

This question is specifically targeting the diagnosis of patellofemoral syndrome. Patients with patellofemoral disorders classically report pain with prolonged knee flexion, and pain relief with knee extension. The "movie theater sign"—in which the patient complains of aching knee pain while sitting with the knees flexed in the theater for a prolonged period of time—is classic for patellofemoral syndrome. Often, to relieve the pain, the patient will report extending the leg into the aisle.

5. **What is the quality of your pain (sharp, shooting, dull, etc.)?**

The answer to this question is most useful for gathering a general gestalt for the patient's complaint. It may not add any specific diagnostic utility, but it will give a better overall picture for the patient's problem.

6. Have you tried anything to help the pain and, if yes, has that been successful?

This question is more useful for when you are contemplating diagnostic tests and treatment strategies.

7. Other important questions to remember to ask include: Have you ever had surgery on your knee? Do you have any hip or ankle pain (both hip and ankle pain can refer pain to the knee, and vice versa)?

Physical Exam

Having completed the history portion of your clinical exam, you are ready for the physical examination.

Observe the patient's gait as the patient walks back and forth across the room. Is the gait antalgic (does the patient favor one leg over the other)? This may not actually help you with the diagnosis, but it will help you gage the degree of impairment, guide what imaging studies to order, and help form your ultimate treatment plan.

With the patient seated, fully extend the patient's knee and determine the quadricep (Q)-angle. The Q-angle is formed by drawing an imaginary line from the anterior superior iliac spine to the center of the patella. This line is intersected by a second line from the tibial tuberosity to the center of the patella and continues superiorly along the center of the anterior thigh (Photo 1). The intersection of these two lines is called the *Q-angle*. A normal Q-angle in males is 10–15°, and in females it is 10–19°. Do not split hairs over angles. After examining several knees, you will begin to get a feel for a "normal" Q-angle and appreciate an abnormal angle. An abnormal Q-angle reflects abnormal patellar tracking and suggests an underlying patellofemoral disorder.

Next, flex and extend the patient's leg and note the tracking of the patella. Excessive lateral tracking is another indication of patellofemoral syndrome. Palpate under and around the patella with the knee in full extension (the knee must be in extension to allow palpation under the surface of the patella). Tenderness in this region is indicative of patellofemoral syndrome.

Then, flex and extend the patient's leg with one hand and palpate the patient's knee joint with the other hand. Crepitus may be an incidental finding, but it is also consistent with osteoarthritis and patellofemoral syndrome.

Next, palpate the patient's tibial tubercle. Pain and tenderness at the tibial tubercle in young individuals is consistent with Osgood-

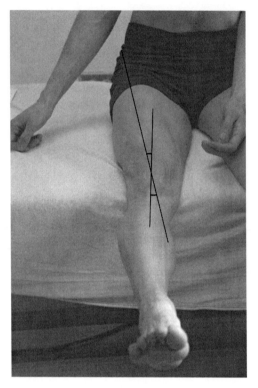

Photo 1. Q-angle.

Schlatter's syndrome. Palpate posteromedial to the tibial tubercle approximately 2 inches below the joint line (Photo 2). This area is the pes anserinus, and it is the point at which the tendons of the sartorius, gracilis, and semitendinosus muscles attach to the tibia. These muscles can be remembered by the convenient pneumonic: Say Grace Before Tea. A bursa overlies the insertion of these tendons and can become inflamed. Tenderness at this point reflects inflammation in the bursa.

While the patient is still seated with legs hanging off the examining table, palpate the patient's joint line between the femoral condyles and tibial plateau. Tenderness along the medial joint line suggests an injury of the medial meniscus or medial collateral ligament. Tenderness along the lateral joint line suggests a lateral meniscus or lateral collateral ligament injury.

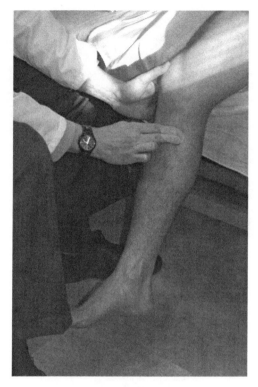

Photo 2. Pes anserinus palpation.

Next, palpate the popliteal fossa and appreciate the pulsation of the popliteal artery. A small swelling in the fossa may indicate a Baker's cyst.

Following this, test the muscles of the patient's knee by having the patient extend the knee against resistance (Photo 3). This tests the quadriceps, which are innervated by the femoral nerve (L2–L4).

Next, have the patient bring the ankle underneath the table (flexing the knee) against resistance (Photo 4). This tests the patient's hamstring muscles, which are innervated primarily by the tibial portion of the sciatic nerve (L5, S1). The common peroneal portion of the sciatic nerve (L5–S2) innervates the short head of the biceps femoris.

Table 1 lists the major movements of the knee, along with the involved muscles and their innervation.

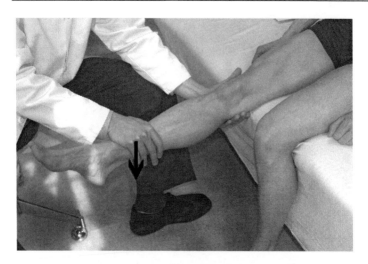

Photo 3. Knee extension against resistance.

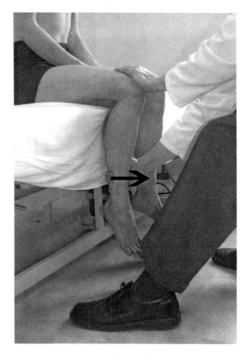

Photo 4. Knee flexion against resistance.

Table 1
Primary Muscles and Innervation for Knee Movement

Major muscle movement	Primary muscles involved	Primary innervation
Knee flexion	Hamstrings (semimembranosus, semitendinosus, biceps femoris).	Primarily tibial, but also peroneal portion of sciatic nerve (primarily L5).
Knee extension	Quadriceps (vastus lateralis, vastus medialis, vastus intermedius, rectus femoris).	Femoral nerve (primarily L4).

Next, test the patellar reflex (L4).

With the patient still seated, test for stability of the medial collateral ligament (MCL). Do this by flexing the patient's knee to 30°. Next, secure the patient's ankle in one hand and cup the patient's knee with the other hand so that your thenar eminence is against the patient's fibular head. Place a firm valgus stress on the patient's knee by pushing medially against the patient's knee and pulling laterally against the patient's ankle—this maneuver is performed in an attempt to open the medial side of his knee (Photo 5). If there is an MCL injury, there will be medial joint-line gapping that you will appreciate with the fingers that are cupped around the patient's knee. When the valgus stress on the patient's leg is relieved, the patient's knee may be felt to "clunk" back together if there is an MCL tear.

To test for a lateral collateral ligament (LCL) tear, apply a varus stress to the patient's joint by pushing the patient's ankle medially while pulling the patient's knee laterally. Remember to keep your hand cupped around the lateral aspect of the joint in order to appreciate gapping, if present (Photo 6). MCL injuries are much more common than LCL injuries.

Next, have the patient lie in the supine position while you check for an effusion. Look for a large effusion by pushing the patient's patella superiorly and then quickly releasing it. If there is a large amount of fluid, the fluid will redistribute and push the patella into its former position. If this happens, it is called a *ballotable patella*. A ballotable patella is a sign of a major effusion. To check for a smaller effusion,

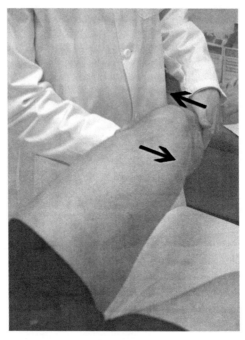

Photo 5. Valgus stress to test the medial collateral ligament.

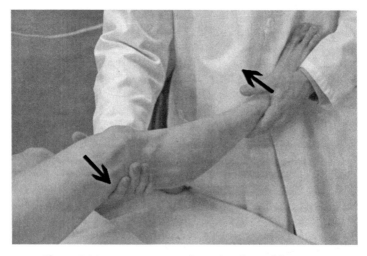

Photo 6. Varus stress to test lateral collateral ligament.

you may need to milk the fluid from the suprapatellar pouch and the lateral side of the knee over to the medial side of the knee. Then, you would release the fluid and tap the medial aspect of the knee. In the next few seconds, if an effusion is present, then the fluid will redistribute laterally and a fullness will develop on the lateral side of the knee.

Now, test for an anterior cruciate ligament (ACL) tear. The most *sensitive* clinical test for an ACL tear is the Lachman test. The Lachman test is performed by flexing the patient's knee to 20° and stabilizing the patient's femur with one hand and pulling the tibia toward you with the other hand. First, test the normal leg to establish the baseline endpoint. This is important because a few degrees of anterior glide of the tibia on the femur may be normal. Next, test the pathologic leg. Increased glide or a loose endpoint suggests an ACL tear.

The anterior drawer test is a similar test that should also be performed to evaluate for an ACL injury. In this test, the patient's knee is flexed to 90° with the feet flat on the table. The examiner sits on the patient's foot to stabilize it, and with the examiner's hands cupped around the back of the patient's upper calf, the tibia is pulled toward the examiner (Photo 7). If the tibia slides forward from under the femur more than a few degrees, there may be a tear in the ACL.

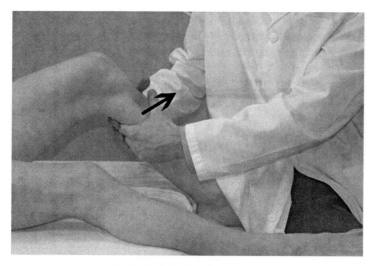

Photo 7. Anterior drawer test.

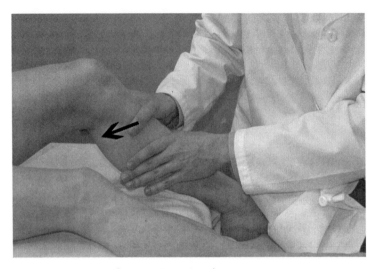

Photo 8. Posterior drawer test.

If the patient has a positive anterior drawer sign or Lachman test, repeat the maneuver with the patient's leg in external and internal rotation. Repeating the maneuver with the leg in external rotation should tighten the posteromedial portion of the capsule. If the patient's tibia glides forward as much as it did with the leg in the neutral position, an MCL tear may be accompanying the potential ACL tear. Repeating the test with the leg in internal rotation tightens the posterolateral capsule. If the patient's tibia again glides forward as much as it did with the leg in the neutral position, an LCL tear may be accompanying the potential ACL tear.

To test for a posterior cruciate ligament (PCL) tear, the examiner stays seated on the patient's foot as for the anterior drawer test. However, instead of pulling the patient's tibia toward the examiner, the tibia is pushed posteriorly (Photo 8). If the patient's tibia glides posteriorly on the femur, it is likely torn, although the PCL is rarely torn. The posterior sag sign is also used to evaluate for a PCL injury. In this sign, the patient's hip is flexed to 45° and the knee is flexed to 90°. The examiner supports the limb by holding the patient's ankle (Photo 9). In a patient with a PCL tear, the tibia will posteriorly translate on the femur.

A torn meniscus is a common injury. Tenderness to palpation at the joint line (which you have already assessed) is a good indication that

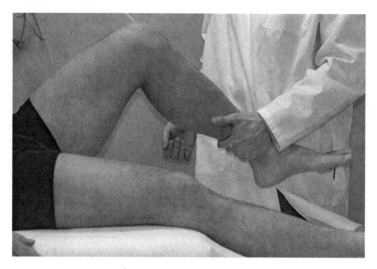

Photo 9. Posterior sag sign.

the meniscus is injured. A few special tests are very useful to further investigate the menisci. The McMurray test was designed to diagnose a tear in the posterior medial meniscus because the posterior horn of the medial meniscus is difficult to palpate. To perform the McMurray test, the examiner instructs the patient to lie supine with legs extended. The examiner then takes hold of the patient's heel and fully flexes the leg. Using the ankle as a fulcrum, the examiner rotates the patient's leg internally and externally to loosen up the knee joint. With the knee joint loose and fully flexed, the examiner continues to use the ankle as a fulcrum and puts the leg into external rotation at the same time as the examiner uses the other hand to push the patient's knee medially, applying a valgus stress. The examiner then slowly extends the knee, maintaining the leg in external rotation and under valgus stress (Photo 10). If this maneuver elicits a palpable or audible click in the patient's knee, the posterior half of the medial meniscus is probably torn.

Another good test to help differentiate between a meniscus tear and a collateral ligament tear is the Apley compression and distraction test. To perform this test, the patient is instructed to lie in the prone position. The examiner stabilizes the thigh with one hand and flexes the patient's knee to 90° with the other hand. The examiner then applies downward pressure to the patient's heel as the examiner internally and

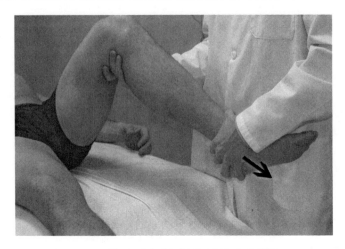

Photo 10. McMurray test.

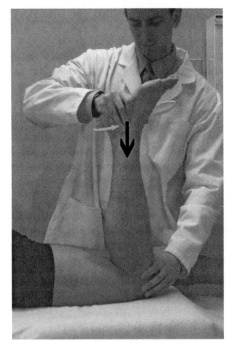

Photo 11. Apley compression test.

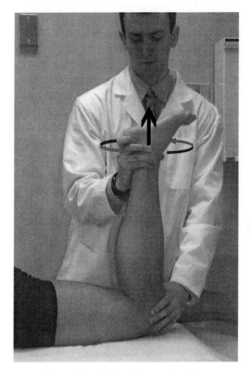

Photo 12. Apley distraction test.

externally rotates the patient's leg (using the patient's heel as the fulcrum) (Photo 11). This is the Apley Compression test. When this maneuver elicits medial pain, the patient may have a medial meniscus or ligament tear. When this maneuver elicits pain on the lateral side, the patient may have a lateral meniscus or ligament tear.

To help differentiate a torn meniscus from a torn ligament, the Apley distraction test is performed next. In the distraction test, the examiner and patient remain in the same position as for the compression test, but in this test the examiner *pulls upward* on the patient's ankle and, still using the ankle as a fulcrum, continues to rotate the patient's leg into internal and external rotation (Photo 12). This maneuver unloads the pressure from the meniscus. Therefore, if this maneuver also elicits pain, the pain is likely coming from an injured ligament and not the meniscus.

Finally, test for osteochondritis dissecans (OCD) of the medial femoral condyle of the knee using Wilson's sign. OCD is a condition in which a fragment of cartilage and subchondral bone separates from an intact articular surface. In the knee, OCD occurs at the medial femoral condyle approximately 80% of the time. To test for Wilson's sign, the examiner has the patient return to lying in the supine position. The examiner takes the patient's knee and ankle and flexes the hip and knee to 90°. Using the patient's ankle as a fulcrum, the examiner internally rotates the leg and then slowly extends the knee (Photo 13). At approximately 30° of flexion, this maneuver most closely abuts the tibial spine against the medial femoral condyle. When this maneuver elicits pain at approximately 30° of flexion, the patient has a positive Wilson's sign. When a positive Wilson's sign is elicited, the examiner next externally

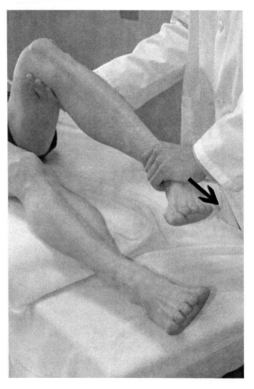

Photo 13. Wilson's sign.

rotates the leg, moving the tibial spine away from the medial femoral condyle. This external rotation should alleviate the patient's pain in a true positive Wilson's sign. If the patient's pain is not alleviated with external rotation, it may be a false positive Wilson's sign.

Plan

Having completed your history and physical examination, you have a good idea of what is wrong with your patient's knee. The following are some general recommendations for what to do next:

- **Suspected ACL tear**

Additional diagnostic evaluation: X-rays, including anteroposterior (AP), lateral, and sunrise views, are taken to rule out fracture. Magnetic resonance imaging (MRI) may be ordered to better delineate the injury.

Treatment: Bracing, nonsteroidal anti-inflammatory drugs (NSAIDs), and physical therapy emphasizing strengthening and stretching the quadriceps and hamstrings, is first-line treatment. Depending on the extent of injury, surgical reconstruction may be necessary.

- **Suspected PCL tear**

Additional diagnostic evaluation: X-rays, including AP, lateral, and sunrise views, should be obtained. MRI may be ordered to delineate the injury.

Treatment: First-line treatment includes rest, ice, physical therapy emphasizing quadriceps strengthening and stretching, and bracing. Depending on the extent of injury, surgery may be required.

- **Suspected MCL injury**

Additional diagnostic evaluation: X-rays, including AP and lateral views, should be obtained. MRI may be ordered when an associated injury is suspected.

Treatment: First-line treatment includes rest, ice, elevation of the joint, physical therapy emphasizing stretching and strengthening exercises, bracing, and crutches until weight-bearing is comfortable. Surgery is rarely necessary.

- **Suspected LCL injury**

Additional diagnostic evaluation: X-rays, including AP and lateral views, should be obtained. MRI may also be helpful.

Treatment: First-line treatment includes rest, ice, NSAIDs, and physical therapy emphasizing stretching and strengthening the quadriceps. Surgery may be required depending on the extent of injury.

- **Suspected meniscus tear**

Additional diagnostic evaluation: X-rays, including AP weight-bearing, AP in 45° extension, lateral, and sunrise views, should be obtained. MRI should also be obtained to better evaluate the extent of injury. Arthroscopy is the gold standard diagnostic tool for meniscal tears but may not be necessary.

Treatment: Small tears may be treated conservatively with rest, ice, bracing, and physical therapy. Larger tears and tears in patients who are competitive athletes and wish to return to competitive sport may require surgery.

- **Suspected patellofemoral disorder**

Additional diagnostic evaluation: X-rays, including AP, lateral, and sunrise views, should be obtained.

Treatment: Rest, NSAIDs, patellar bracing and/or taping, and physical therapy that emphasizes quadriceps stretching and strengthening and straight leg-raising with the leg externally rotated to particularly focus on the vastus medialis oblique, is first-line treatment. Surgery should be reserved for patients who fail to respond to at least several months of aggressive conservative care.

- **Suspected osteoarthritis**

Additional diagnostic evaluation: X-rays, including AP, lateral, sunrise, and posteroanterior views with the knee flexed to 45°, should be obtained.

Treatment: Conservative care, including rest, weight loss (when appropriate), physical therapy—including nonimpact exercises, such as swimming—acetaminophen, NSAIDs, heat modalities, activity modification, ambulatory aids, such as a cane, should be used. Topical analgesic therapy with methylsalicylate or capsaicin cream may be beneficial. Oral glucosamine sulfate (1500 mg) and chondroitin sulfate (1200 mg) taken daily are also helpful. Intra-articular injections of hyaluronic acid improve symptoms temporarily but typically need to be repeated periodically (about once every 6 months). Intra-articular injections of corticosteroid and anesthetic may also be helpful. Surgical options are reserved for persistent or severe symptoms and include arthroscopy, osteotomy, and total knee replacement.

- **Suspected prepatellar bursitis**

  Additional diagnostic evaluation: X-rays, including AP and lateral views, may be obtained to rule out a more serious underlying process.
  Treatment: NSAIDs, activity modification, knee pads, and a corticosteroid and anesthetic injection may be helpful.

- **Suspected pes anserine bursitis**

  Additional diagnostic evaluation: X-rays, including AP and lateral views, may be obtained to rule out a more serious underlying disorder.
  Treatment: NSAIDs, rest, activity modification, physical therapy emphasizing stretching and strengthening of the hamstrings and quadriceps and a corticosteroid and anesthetic injection may be helpful.

- **Suspected OCD**

  Additional diagnostic evaluation: X-rays, including AP and lateral views, and MRI should be obtained.
  Treatment: Conservative care includes physical therapy and bracing. Depending on the age of the patient and extent of injury, surgery may be necessary. Adults generally require surgery, whereas children and adolescents with skeletally immature bones may be treated conservatively.

- **Suspected Osgood-Schlatter's disease**

  Additional diagnostic evaluation: X-rays, including AP and lateral views, may be obtained.
  Treatment: Activity restriction and/or modification, an infrapatellar strap, and physical therapy emphasizing stretching and strengthening of the quadriceps and hamstrings, are generally sufficient for treatment.

7 Ankle Pain

First Thoughts

When a patient complains of "ankle pain," without hearing another word your differential diagnosis includes the following three common etiologies:

1. Ligament injury.
2. Achilles tendonitis.
3. Ankle fracture.

Less common problems that you must still consider include capsular injury, posterior tibial tendonitis, tarsal tunnel syndrome, osteochondritis dissecans (OCD), and anterior impingement syndrome. The history and physical examination will help you narrow your differential diagnosis.

History

Ask the following questions:

1. Where is your pain?

This is a high-yield question. Lateral pain suggests a ligament injury or a possible fracture. Medial pain suggests a ligament injury (rare on the medial side), possible fracture, or posterior tibial tendonitis. Anterior pain suggests anterior capsule injury or anterior bony impingement. Posterior pain suggests Achilles tendinitis. OCD may occur on the lateral or medial aspect of the ankle, but it is a relatively uncommon disorder.

2. When did your pain begin and what were you doing at the time?

This is another high-yield question. In fact, between knowing the location of the patient's pain and how the pain started, you may be

From: *Pocket Guide to Musculoskeletal Diagnosis*
G. Cooper

able to diagnose the pathology of many, if not most, of your patients with ankle pain before even laying hands or eyes on their ankles. Almost all ankle sprains are lateral sprains and occur after an inversion injury. The typical history a patient will give is falling over a turned-in (inverted) ankle while playing a sport or walking in the street.

However, if the patient suffered an ankle fracture, he or she will give a history of a more significant trauma, such as participation in a sporting event in which another player fell on the ankle. If the patient has an anterior capsular strain, the patient may be a softball or baseball player who was injured during a hook-slide into a base. If the patient has Achilles tendonitis, he or she may be a runner, dancer, or other athlete who complains of gradually increasing pain in the Achilles tendon that is made worse with activity. If the patient has posterior tibial tendonitis, the patient is probably a young runner who presents with a complaint of pain at the medial aspect of the ankle with weight-bearing. The patient will report that the pain is worse in the morning and also increases with activity. If the patient has anterior bony impingement syndrome, the patient may be a dancer or basketball player who recalls a history of trauma leading to acute pain followed by chronic, vague pain that is made worse on landing from jumps.

3. Do you experience any locking or catching in your ankle?

This question most directly focuses on OCD. Patients with ankle OCD may have locking and/or catching. OCD is a condition in which a fragment of cartilage and subchondral bone separates from an intact articular surface. In contrast to OCD in other parts of the body, ankle OCD is more typically precipitated by a traumatic insult.

4. Have you ever had surgery on your ankle?

This question is important for many reasons including that patients with a history of ankle surgery are predisposed to premature osteoarthritis in the ankle.

5. What is the quality of your ankle pain (sharp, shooting, dull, aching, burning)?

Patients with tarsal tunnel syndrome may have shooting pains, tingling, and burning radiating from the tarsal tunnel (posterior to the medial malleolus) to the sole of the foot. The answer to this question is also useful for obtaining a gestalt of the patient's pain.

6. **Other questions include: Is there anything you have done for your ankle that has helped the pain? Are you able to bear weight on your ankle?**

These questions are more important for when you consider what imaging studies to order and what treatment to offer the patient.

Physical Exam

Having completed taking your patient's history, you are ready to perform your physical exam.

Observe the patient walking back and forth in the examining room. Is the gait antalgic (i.e., is the patient limping)? Is the patient able to bear weight on the ankle? The patient's weight-bearing status is more important for prognosis, imaging, and treatment considerations than it is for diagnosis, but it should be noted.

Have the patient sit down on the examining table. After an initial survey of the patient's ankles for symmetry and swelling, take the affected ankle in your hand. With your fingers, trace the tibia inferiorly until it ends in the medial malleolus. Palpate the strong medial collateral ligament (MCL; deltoid ligament) that is just inferior to the medial malleolus. Note that this strong ligament is harder to palpate than its lateral counterparts. Tenderness over the MCL may indicate a ligamentous tear from an eversion injury.

Next, move your fingers to the soft tissue depression between the medial malleolus and the calcaneus (heel). The tarsal tunnel is in this depression. The tendons of the flexor hallucis longus muscle, flexor digitorum longus muscle, tibialis posterior muscle, the posterior tibial artery, and posterior tibial nerve run in the tarsal tunnel. Check for the posterior tibial artery's pulse.

To accentuate the tibialis posterior tendon, have the patient invert and plantarflex the foot. Tenderness over this tendon may reflect tibialis posterior tendonitis (Photo 1). Also, check for tibialis posterior tendonitis at its origin in the medial superior half of the tibia. This disorder is sometimes termed "shin splints." To check for this disorder, have the patient invert the foot against resistance. When this maneuver elicits pain along the proximal or middle tibia, the patient may have tibialis posterior tendonitis. When the patient localizes the pain with resisted inversion to the posterior medial malleolus, the patient may have tibialis posterior tendonitis at the point of pain elicitation.

To evaluate for tarsal tunnel syndrome, check for a positive Tinel's sign. To elicit this sign, the tarsal tunnel is repetitively tapped. When

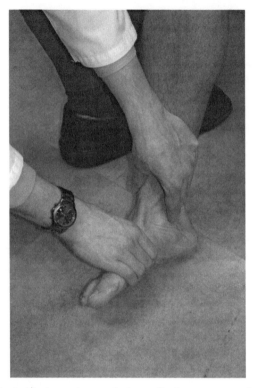

Photo 1. Ankle inversion and plantarflexion accentuating the tibialis posterior tendon.

this tapping elicits radiating pain, burning, numbness, and/or tingling in the distribution of the posterior tibial nerve along the medial malleolus and/or sole of the foot, the sign is positive and indicates that the patient may have tarsal tunnel syndrome. Manual compression of the nerve at the tarsal tunnel for 60 seconds is also used to diagnose tarsal tunnel syndrome (Photo 2). When compression of the nerve for 60 seconds reproduces your patient's symptoms, the test is positive for tarsal tunnel syndrome.

Now, move your fingers to the posterior ankle and palpate the large Achilles tendon (this is the thickest and strongest tendon in the body). Tenderness over the Achilles tendon implicates Achilles tendonitis as the source of pain. Trace the Achilles tendon inferiorly and note

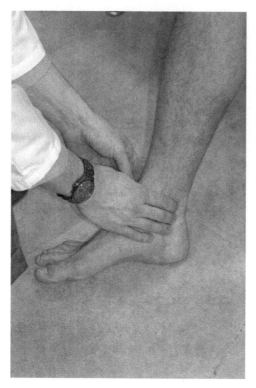

Photo 2. Tarsal tunnel compression.

the insertion of the Achilles tendon into the calcaneus. A bursa lies between the anterior surface of the Achilles tendon and the calcaneus. Another bursa lies between the insertion of the Achilles tendon and the overlying skin. Either of these two bursae may become inflamed and cause pain. Tenderness over the bursa implicates bursitis as the cause of pain. These bursae are discussed more fully in Chapter 8.

If the patient has complained of trauma to the Achilles tendon or a sudden exertion in which pushing off from the patient's toes resulted in severe pain, swelling, and weakness in the calf, then the patient may have ruptured the Achilles tendon. If a defect in the Achilles tendon is present, you may be able to palpate it. Another good test for a rupture of the Achilles tendon is to have the patient lie in the prone position with the patient's legs dangling off the edge of the examining table. Next,

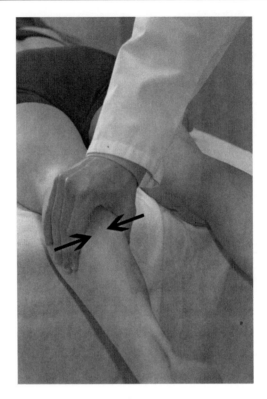

Photo 3. Thompson test.

squeeze the patient's calf (Photo 3). If the foot fails to plantarflex or only partly plantarflexes, the patient probably has a ruptured Achilles tendon. This maneuver is called the Thompson test.

Test the muscles of the ankle by first having the patient dorsiflex the foot against resistance (Photo 4). This tests the tibialis anterior muscle, which is innervated by the deep peroneal nerve (L4).

Next, have the patient plantarflex the foot against resistance (Photo 5). This tests the patient's gastrocneumius and soleus muscles, which are innervated by the tibial nerve (primarily S1).

Then, test the Achilles reflex (S1).

Assess the integrity of the ligaments of the patient's ankle joint. The anterior talofibular ligament (ATFL) attaches from the anterior portion of the lateral malleolus to the lateral aspect of the talar neck in the

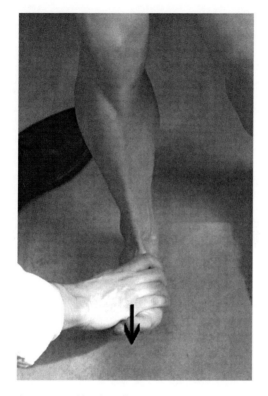

Photo 4. Ankle dorsiflexion against resistance.

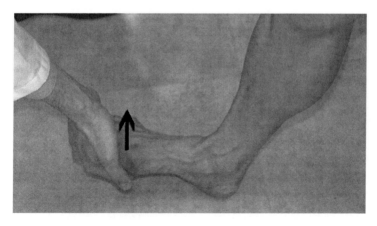

Photo 5. Ankle plantarflexion against resistance.

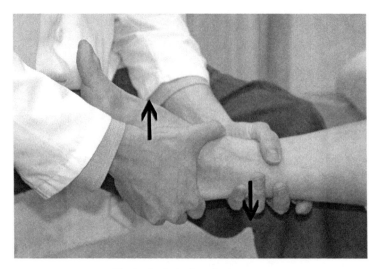

Photo 6. Anterior drawer test.

foot. The ATFL is the most commonly sprained ankle ligament in part because it is the first to be stressed during inversion and plantar flexion. To test the ATFL, first check for ATFL tenderness. Next, put the ankle into plantar flexion and inversion. If this causes pain, the ATFL is probably injured. To further test the ATFL, perform the anterior drawer test. To perform this test, with the patient's foot in a few degrees of plantar flexion, take hold of the patient's lower tibia with one hand and grip the patient's calcaneus with the palm of the other hand. Pull the patient's calcaneus (and talus) anteriorly toward you while you simultaneously push the patient's tibia posteriorly away from you (Photo 6). The ATFL is the only ligament resisting this anterior talar subluxation. Increased subluxation and/or a clunking sensation with subluxation reflect a torn ATFL.

The calcaneofibular ligament (CFL) attaches the fibula to the lateral wall of the calcaneus. The CFL is the second ligament to be torn in an ankle sprain. For an ankle to be unstable, both the ATFL and the CFL must be torn. To test for the integrity of the CFL and ATFL, invert the patient's calcaneus and assess for gapping of the talar joint (Photo 7). Increased gapping (compared with the unaffected limb) indicates a torn ATFL and CFL and reflects ankle instability.

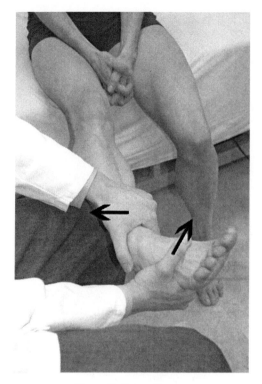

Photo 7. Talar tilt test.

The posterior talofibular ligament (PTFL) is the third ligament in the lateral ankle to be sprained. The PTFL attaches from the posterior edge of the lateral malleolus to the posterior aspect of the talus. Because of its position and strength, the PTFL is rarely torn except in severe ankle injuries, such as dislocation.

Having assessed the integrity of the lateral ligaments, next assess the integrity of the MCL. Stabilize the patient's leg by holding the patient's tibia and calcaneus and evert the foot (Photo 8). Increased gapping at the medial ankle reflects a tear in the medial collateral ligament.

Finally, if you are concerned about a possible stress fracture in the lower leg or foot, place a tuning fork onto the painful area or area of localized tenderness *over the bone*. Vibration causes increased pain in a stress fracture. Confirm your findings with imaging studies (usually X-rays).

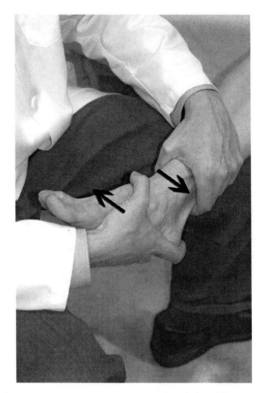

Photo 8. Eversion stress to test the deltoid ligament.

Plan

Having completed your history and physical examination, you have a good idea of what is wrong with your patient's ankle. Here is what to do next:

- **Suspected ankle sprain**

Additional diagnostic evaluation: The Ottawa ankle rules were designed to offer an evidence-based approach to determine which patients with a suspected ankle sprain require X-rays and which do not. All patients with a suspected ankle sprain require radiographs *except* patients who are younger than 55 years old, able to walk four steps at the time of injury and at the time of evaluation, and who do not have tenderness over the posterior edge of the medial malleolus. If the diagnosis is in doubt, or concomitant injury to the soft tissues is suspected, magnetic resonance imaging (MRI) may also be very helpful.

Treatment: most ankle sprains may be managed conservatively with rest, ice, compression, and protective devices, such as an air cast (or other brace). Physical therapy that emphasizes range of motion, proprioceptive, and strengthening exercises is also helpful. Return to sport is governed primarily by symptoms. In general, once a patient can run, jump 10 times on the injured foot, stand for 1 min with eyes closed on the injured foot, and pivot quickly without significant pain, the patient is ready to return to sport. Most ankle sprains do not require surgery. Indications for surgery may include severe MCL sprains.

- **Suspected Achilles tendonitis**

Additional diagnostic evaluation: X-rays, including anteroposterior (AP) and lateral views, may reveal a spur at the Achilles tendon insertion. However, X-rays are not always necessary.

Treatment: Conservative care is first-line therapy and includes rest, orthotics, ice, and physical therapy.

- **Suspected retrocalcaneal bursitis**

See Chapter 8 for discussion.

- **Suspected anterior impingement syndrome**

Additional diagnostic evaluation: None necessary.

Treatment: Conservative care is first-line therapy with ice, rest, nonsteroidal anti-inflammatory drugs (NSAIDs), and physical therapy. Surgery is occasionally necessary.

- **Suspected tarsal tunnel syndrome**

Additional diagnostic evaluation: X-rays, including AP and lateral views, may be obtained to rule out other pathological processes. Electrodiagnostic studies may be used to confirm the diagnosis.

Treatment: Rest, ice, NSAIDs, lidocaine patch, and/or a steroid and anesthetic injection are helpful. Surgical release is reserved for severe cases that are not responsive to conservative care.

- **Suspected osteoarthritis**

Additional diagnostic evaluation: X-rays, including standing AP and lateral views, should be obtained.

Treatment: Conservative care, including weight loss, rest, activity modification, nonweight-bearing exercises, acetaminophen, and NSAIDs, may be used. Intra-articular injection of corticosteroid and anesthetic may also be helpful. Surgery is rare and reserved for severe cases that are not responsive to more conservative measures.

- **Suspected Achilles tendon rupture**

Additional diagnostic evaluation: X-rays, including standing AP and lateral views, should be obtained to rule out associated injury. Ultrasound and/or MRI may be obtained to confirm the diagnosis.

Treatment: Surgical repair is often necessary and is recommended for most patients who can tolerate the surgery. Repair is particularly recommended in young and/or active patients wishing to return to an active lifestyle. More conservative measures include bracing. Physical therapy is started after surgical repair or a period of bracing.

- **Suspected ankle fracture**

Ankle fractures include fracture of the medial malleolus, lateral malleolus, or both malleoli. When both malleoli are involved, the fracture is unstable. Associated ligamentous injury may also make the fracture unstable.

Additional diagnostic evaluation: X-rays, including AP, lateral, and mortise views with the foot in 15–20° of rotation, should be obtained. Occasionally bone scan and/or computed tomography may be necessary.

Treatment: If the fracture is stable, casting for 1–2 months may be sufficient. Unstable or displaced fractures require surgical intervention.

8 Foot Pain

First Thoughts

When a patient complains of "foot pain," your differential diagnosis of most common causes is fairly broad and includes fracture, interdigital (Morton's) neuroma, tarsal tunnel syndrome, hallux valgus, hallux rigidus, retrocalcaneal or calcaneal bursitis, sesamoiditis, and plantar fasciitis. Do not be intimidated by the relatively large differential diagnosis. Thankfully, a brief history and physical exam will differentiate most common etiologies of foot pain. In addition, the most common underlying causes of foot pain are generally identifiable and easily corrected. The most common causes are footwear, footwear, and/or footwear. Indeed, most cases of foot pain can be blamed, at least in part, on the ergonomically challenged fashion sensibilities of the modern world: narrow shoes with poor arch supports and small toe-boxes. Luckily, many cases of foot pain can be treated with sensible shoes and quality orthotics.

History

Ask the following questions:

1. Where is your pain?

This high-yield question, in combination with a glance at your patient's footwear, will give you the diagnosis in many cases. If the patient points at the first metatarsophalangeal joint, then the patient probably has hallux rigidus caused, in part, by ill-fitting shoes. If the patient points at the first metatarsocuneiform joint, the patient probably has hallux valgus (bunions) that are usually caused by a small toe-box in the shoe. If the patient points to the second or third interdigital space, the patient has an interdigital neuroma that is generally caused by a narrow shoe toe-box. Pain in the metatarsals (particularly the second metatarsal) may be metatarsalgia. If the patient points to the bottom of the foot, the patient may have a stress fracture, tarsal tunnel syndrome, plantar fasciitis, calcaneal bursitis, or retrocalcaneal bursitis. Pain beneath the first metatarsal head may be sesamoiditis. Pain at the ball of the foot may be a contusion or stress fracture of one of the sesamoid bones. Further questioning will help distinguish these disorders.

2. How and when did your pain begin?

If the patient has plantar fasciitis, the patient will give a history of insidious onset of *medial* plantar heel pain that begins on taking the first step of the morning. Classically, the pain alleviates after a few steps but tends to return later in the evening.

Patients with sesamoiditis complain of pain that began or became more pronounced during jumping or pushing off to run. Patients with calcaneal or retrocalcaneal bursitis may complain of pain with running. Patients with stress fractures complain of progressively worsening pain that usually is precipitated by an increase in activity intensity. For example, if the patient begins training for a marathon and is running more than usual, the patient may develop a stress fracture. Patients with an interdigital neuroma, metatarsalgia, hallux valgus, or hallux rigidus may complain of pain that began with a change in footwear. The pain will be worse after wearing the new shoes for a whole day. An insidious onset of intractable heel pain is indicative of tarsal tunnel syndrome.

3. What is the quality of your pain (e.g., sharp, dull, aching, burning, electric)?

Patients with tarsal tunnel syndrome will complain of numbness and burning in addition to pain behind the medial malleolus and at the sole of the foot.

4. Other important questions to ask include: What makes the pain better or worse? Are you able to bear weight? These questions are most helpful when deciding on imaging studies and treatment.

Physical Exam

Having completed taking your patient's history, you are ready to perform your physical exam.

Instruct the patient to stand barefoot in front of you. Note any asymmetry in the arches of the feet. Next, palpate the patient's foot beginning with the first digit (hallux). Instruct the patient to dorsiflex as you dorsally palpate the first digit. Tenderness with this maneuver indicates an underlying sesamoiditis. Tenderness and decreased range of motion of the first metatarsalphalangeal (MTP) joint may indicate hallux rigidus. Pain elicited by resisted plantarflexion of the first digit may indicate flexor hallucis longus tenosynovitis. Tenderness to palpation over the fifth MTP indicates a Jones fracture, until proven oth-erwise with radiographs.

Squeezing the metatarsal bones together while simultaneously palpating a painful web space is the compression test for interdigital neuroma. If an interdigital neuroma is present, the involved web space should be tender to palpation with this maneuver.

Allow the patient's history to further guide your physical examination. Palpate the bones of the foot, paying particular attention to any painful areas. Tenderness over a bone may indicate a stress fracture. Place a vibrating tuning fork over the bony tender spot. Stress fractures will have increased pain with vibration. Palpate the calcaneal and retrocalcaneal bursae (Photo 1). Tenderness over one of the bursae indicates a bursitis.

Tarsal tunnel syndrome may cause pain, tingling, burning, and/or numbness in the sole of the foot. This exam and the management of this syndrome are discussed in Chapter 7.

Passive dorsiflexion will stretch the plantar fascia and pain with this maneuver reveals plantar fasciitis (Photo 2). Medial heel tenderness at the plantar fascia attachments may also indicate plantar fasciitis.

Part of the physical examination of a patient with foot pain includes examining the patient's footwear. As you examine the footwear, ask yourself the following questions: are the shoes causing the foot pain? Note the size of the toe-box. Is there enough room for the toes? Is there enough of an arch support for the patient's feet? Is one side of the shoe being worn down more than normal? Would orthotics be helpful for this patient?

Plan

Having completed your history and physical examination, you have a good idea of what is causing your patient's foot pain. Here is what to do next:

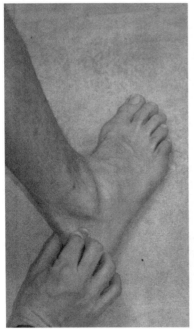

Photo 1. Calcaneal and retrocal-   Photo 2. Passive dorsiflexion.
caneal bursa palpation.

- **Suspected metatarsalgia**

Additional diagnostic evaluation: X-rays, including standing anteroposterior (AP) and lateral views, should be obtained to rule out fracture.

Treatment: Metatarsal pads are very effective. Shoes with a wider toe-box and good arch support may also be helpful.

- **Suspected hallux valgus (bunion)**

Additional diagnostic evaluation: X-rays, including standing AP and lateral views, should be obtained.

Treatment: Conservative care includes shoes with a wide toe-box and orthotics. Surgical excision of the deformity is reserved for severe cases that do not respond to conservative care.

- **Suspected retrocalcaneal bursitis**

  Additional diagnostic evaluation: X-rays, including standing AP and lateral views, may be obtained.

  Treatment: Conservative care, including Achilles tendon stretching, activity modification, and orthotics, is usually successful. Surgical treatment is reserved for severe cases resistant to conservative care.

- **Suspected Morton's neuroma**

  Additional diagnostic evaluation: None necessary.

  Treatment: Conservative treatment is the initial management and may include rest, a metatarsal pad, and/or a corticosteroid and anesthetic injection. Surgical nerve excision is reserved for severe cases that do not respond to more conservative treatment.

- **Suspected plantar fasciitis**

  Additional diagnostic evaluation: None necessary.

  Treatment: Conservative care is usually adequate and includes rest, passive stretching, ice and/or heat, and nonsteroidal anti-inflammatory drugs (NSAIDs). A corticosteroid and anesthetic injection may also be helpful. Surgical endoscopic plantar fascia release is reserved for severe or recalcitrant symptoms.

- **Suspected tarsal tunnel syndrome**

  Discussed in Chapter 7.

- **Suspected flexor hallucis longis tenosynovitis**

  Additional diagnostic evaluation: X-rays, including standing AP and lateral views, may be helpful. Magnetic resonance imaging (MRI) and/or ultrasound may be used to rule out associated pathology and evaluate the extent of injury.

  Treatment: Conservative care includes rest, ice, activity modification, and NSAIDs. Surgical release is rarely necessary.

- **Suspected Jones fracture (fifth metatarsal fracture)**

  Additional diagnostic evaluation: X-rays, including AP, lateral, and oblique views, should be obtained.

Treatment: Casting for 6 to 8 weeks and nonweight-bearing status is used to treat some Jones fractures. Surgery may be necessary for intra-articular tuberosity fractures.

- **Suspected stress fracture**

Additional diagnostic evaluation: X-rays, including AP, lateral, and oblique views, should be obtained, but it must be remembered that X-rays may not show changes for up to 3 weeks after a stress fracture. Bone scan and MRI may help confirm the diagnosis and may be positive as little as 2 days after stress fracture.

Treatment: Nondisplaced fractures (except in the case of a Jones fracture, navicular bone, or other high-risk location fracture) may generally be treated with rest, ice, orthotics, and a walking cast. Displaced fractures (or fractures in a high-risk location) generally require surgery.

Index

Lightning Source UK Ltd.
Milton Keynes UK
UKOW050007221111

182440UK00001B/127/P